TRALI:
Mechanisms, Management, and Prevention

Editors

Steven Kleinman, MD
University of British Columbia School of Medicine
Vancouver, British Columbia, Canada

Mark A. Popovsky, MD
Harvard Medical School
Boston, Massachusetts
and
Haemonetics Corporation
Braintree, Massachusetts

AABB Press
Bethesda, MD
2008

AABB
8101 Glenbrook Road
Bethesda, Maryland 20814-2749

ISBN 978-1-56395-267-8
Printed in the United States

Library of Congress Cataloging-in-Publication Data

TRALI : mechanisms, management, and prevention / editors, Steven Kleinman, Mark A. Popovsky.
   p. ; cm.
Includes bibliographical references and index.
ISBN 978-1-56395-267-8
  1. Respiratory distress syndrome. 2. Lungs—Wounds and injuries. 3. Blood—Transfusion—Complications.
I. Kleinman, Steven. II. Popovsky, Mark A., 1950- III. AABB. IV. Title: Transfusion-related acute lung injury.
  [DNLM: 1. Respiratory Distress Syndrome, Adult—physiopathology. 2. Respiratory Distress Syndrome,
Adult—prevention & control. 3. Blood Transfusion—adverse effects. 4. Blood Transfusion—standards. WF
140 T769 2008]
  RC776.R38T73 2008
  616.2'4—dc22
                        2008035795

Contributors

Richard J. Benjamin, MD, PhD, FRCPath
American Red Cross Blood Services
National Headquarters
Washington, District of Columbia

Jürgen Bux, MD, PhD
German Red Cross Blood Donor
Service West
Hagen, Germany

Rodrigo Cartin-Ceba, MD
Mayo Clinic
Rochester, Minnesota

Catherine E. Chapman, BSc, MD, FRCP, FRCPath
National Health Service Blood and
Transplant (Newcastle Blood Centre)
Newcastle, United Kingdom

Anne F. Eder, MD, PhD
American Red Cross Blood Services
National Headquarters
Washington, District of Columbia

Ognjen Gajic, MD, MSc
Mayo Clinic
Rochester, Minnesota

Hasrat Khan, MD
MeritCare Medical Center
Fargo, North Dakota

Steven Kleinman, MD
University of British Columbia School
of Medicine
Vancouver, Canada

Patricia M. Kopko, MD
BloodSource
Mather, California

Mark R. Looney, MD
Division of Pulmonary and Critical
Care Medicine
University of California
San Francisco, California

Mark A. Popovsky, MD
Harvard Medical School
Boston, Massachusetts
Haemonetics Corporation
Braintree, Massachusetts

Ulrich J.H. Sachs, MD, PhD
Institute for Clinical Immunology
and Transfusion Medicine
Justus Liebig University
Giessen, Germany

David F. Stroncek, MD
Warren G. Magnuson Clinical Center
National Institutes of Health
Bethesda, Maryland

Pearl Toy, MD
Blood Bank and Donor Center
University of California
San Francisco, California

Darrell Triulzi, MD
Institute for Transfusion Medicine
University of Pittsburgh
School of Medicine
Pittsburgh, Pennsylvania

Lorna M. Williamson, BSc, MD, FRCP, FRCPath
University of Cambridge
National Health Service Blood
and Transplant
Cambridge, United Kingdom

Table of Contents

*Mark A. Popovsky, MD; Pearl Toy, MD; and
Mark R. Looney, MD*

*Hasrat Khan, MD; Rodrigo Cartin-Ceba, MD; and
Ognjen Gajic, MD, MSc*

Preface

THE SYNDROME NOW RECOGNIZED AS TRANS-fusion-related acute lung injury (TRALI) certainly existed before its first description in 1985. Several individual or small cluster case reports of a transfusion reaction similar to acute respiratory distress syndrome had appeared in the literature since 1951 under different descriptors—allergic pulmonary edema, leukoagglutinin transfusion reaction, pulmonary hypersensitivity reaction, or noncardiogenic pulmonary edema. The clinical descriptions in each of these entities are consistent with the definition of TRALI that has been in use since the 2004 Canadian Consensus Conference. Acute hypoxemia and acute pulmonary edema in the setting of transfusion are the hallmarks of TRALI.

From 1985 until the early to mid-1990s, relatively little attention was paid to TRALI, probably because of the misperception that the lung was not an important target of posttransfusion injury. That perception changed as scores of reports and studies were published that underscored the fact that this was a condition with significant morbidity and high mortality. When TRALI surpassed all other causes of death from transfusion in the United States and the United Kingdom, the medical community began to take notice in earnest. Hemovigilance systems in Canada and France have confirmed the importance of TRALI. Today there is general agreement that in countries with high human development indexes, TRALI is the most important cause of morbidity and mortality from transfusion. In addition, the study of TRALI has increased awareness of other complications of transfusion that affect the lung, most importantly circulatory overload.

Coincident with the morbidity data, studies of epidemiology and pathophysiology have appeared and have advanced knowledge of the triggering factors and the pathways that lead to the respiratory distress syndrome. The association of TRALI with plasma-containing components from multiparous female donors (in some cases with demonstrated leukocyte antibodies) is important and has significant implications for blood collectors. Strategies to identify "high-risk" donors are being developed and, in some countries, implemented. The issues raised by these strategies are addressed in this book.

One of the reasons that this book has been written is that TRALI has moved beyond the confines of the hospital transfusion service or regional blood collector. The book is intended to provide transfusion medicine professionals, transfusing clinicians, and other health-care staff with an up-to-date reference guide to all the key issues related to TRALI. Each chapter has been written by a recognized authority in the field and is intended to summarize existing knowledge as well as to highlight areas of ongoing discussion and investigation. The goal is to provide an accessible tool that gives both an overview and a detailed picture of the relevant clinical, laboratory, pathophysiologic, and donor-related issues posed by TRALI.

Mark A. Popovsky, MD
Steven Kleinman, MD
Editors

About the Editors

Steven Kleinman, **MD,** is an internationally recognized expert in the field of blood safety. His professional experience has included positions as medical director of a regional blood center (American Red Cross in Southern California, 1982-1991), medical codirector of a transfusion service (University of California, Los Angeles Medical Center, 1991-1995), and investigator in several multicenter transfusion medicine research studies, including the ongoing Retrovirus Epidemiology Donor Study-II, sponsored by the National Heart, Lung, and Blood Institute.

Since 1996, he has been President of a transfusion medicine consulting company (Kleinman Biomedical Research) located in Victoria, British Columbia, whose clients include blood collection organizations, government, and industry in both the United States and Canada. He is also Clinical Professor of Pathology at the University of British Columbia and Senior Medical Advisor to AABB.

Dr. Kleinman has published over 100 peer-reviewed scientific articles and over 20 book chapters, and he has co-edited a textbook in transfusion medicine. He has chaired the AABB Transfusion-Transmitted Disease Committee, the AABB Interagency Task Force on Bacterial Contamination of Platelets, and the Consensus Panel at the Canadian Consensus Conference on TRALI. He currently chairs the AABB TRALI Working Group.

Mark A. Popovsky, MD, is an honors graduate of the University of Vermont College of Medicine. He received his training in anatomic and clinical pathology at the National Institutes of Health, and the Mayo Clinic provided his training in transfusion medicine. He served as Director of the Transfusion and Intravenous Services at the Mayo Clinic from 1982 to 1985. In 1985, he assumed the role of Medical Director of the American Red Cross—New England Region, a position he held until 1995. From 1996 to 2000, he was Chief Executive Officer and Chief Medical Officer of the New England Region.

Dr. Popovsky is an Associate Clinical Professor of Pathology at Harvard Medical School and Beth Israel Deaconess Medical Center in Boston, MA. He has authored or coauthored over 375 publications in transfusion medicine and is the editor of the three editions of the reference book *Transfusion Reactions.*

He currently serves as Vice President and Chief Medical Officer of the Haemonetics Corporation. Dr. Popovsky serves on the editorial boards of five journals and has held positions on numerous AABB national and international committees. He served in Nigeria in 2004 as a member of the US President's Emergency Plan for AIDS Relief delegation to that country. He is the recipient of numerous awards for contributions to transfusion medicine and teaching from institutions including the National Institutes of Health, Massachusetts Association of Blood Banks, University of Iowa, and University of Vermont. He is the 2009 Emily Cooley Lecturer and Awardee.

In: Kleinman S, Popovsky MA, eds.
TRALI: Mechanisms, Management, and Prevention
Bethesda, MD: AABB Press, 2008

1

The Spectrum of Pulmonary Transfusion Reactions

MARK A. POPOVSKY, MD; PEARL TOY, MD; AND
MARK R. LOONEY, MD

IF, WITH RESPECT TO THE COMPLICATIONS OF transfusion, the 1980s was the "AIDS era," it may be said that the first decade of the 21st century is the "pulmonary era." Indeed, the lung as the target organ of transfusion-induced injury has emerged from being considered inconsequential to being the foremost problem today in many countries. This chapter considers the clinical

Mark A. Popovsky, MD, Associate Clinical Professor, Harvard Medical School, Boston, Massachusetts, and Vice President and Chief Medical Officer, Haemonetics Corporation, Braintree, Massachusetts; Pearl Toy, MD, Professor, Department of Laboratory Medicine, and Chief, Blood Bank and Donor Center, University of California, San Francisco, California; and Mark R. Looney, MD, Assistant Professor of Medicine, Division of Pulmonary and Critical Care Medicine, University of California, San Francisco, California aspects of the major pulmonary complications associated with transfusion.

Transfusion-related acute lung injury (TRALI) was first recognized as a syndrome in the 1980s. Case reports of acute pulmonary edema in the absence of myocardial injury or circulatory overload appeared as early as 1951 and infrequently into the 1970s.[1-4] Such reactions were labeled with a variety of terms, such as "noncardiogenic edema," "allergic pulmonary edema," "leukoagglutinin transfusion reaction," and "hypersensitivity reaction."[2-4] Popovsky and Moore first defined TRALI as acute pulmonary edema, respiratory distress, hypoxemia, hypotension, and fever in the setting of a recent plasma-containing transfusion.[5]

Definitions

TRALI is a form of acute lung injury (ALI). The North American-European Consensus Conference defined ALI as acute hypoxemia with a partial pressure of oxygen in arterial blood/inspired oxygen concentration (PaO_2/FiO_2) ratio of <300 mm Hg with bilateral pulmonary edema on a frontal chest radiograph.[6] Additionally, either the pulmonary artery occlusion pressure is <18 mm Hg, or there is no clinical evidence of left atrial hypertension. Recognized risk factors for ALI include sepsis, pneumonia, aspiration of gastric contents, pancreatitis, burns, drug overdose, disseminated intravascular coagulation, fracture of long bones, near drowning, and massive transfusion.[4,5]

Two recently published definitions of TRALI are presented in Table 1-1.[4,6-8] These definitions rely on the North American-European Consensus Conference definition of ALI. Both definitions consider instances of new ALI within 6 hours of transfusion—in the absence of other risk factors for ALI—as TRALI. The National Heart, Lung, and Blood Institute (NHLBI) Working Group and the Canadian Consensus Conference differ with respect to ALI within 6 hours of transfusion in the presence of risk factors for ALI. The Canadian Consensus Conference de-

Table 1-1. Definitions of TRALI*

Patients without an Alternative Risk Factor for ALI	Patients with an Alternative Risk Factor for ALI	
Definition	Canadian Consensus Conference Definition	NHLBI Working Group Definition

• New ALI:
  – Acute onset
  – Hypoxemia—$PaO_2/FiO_2 \le 300$ mm Hg or O_2 sat ≤90% on room air
  – Bilateral infiltrates on frontal chest radiograph
  – No evidence of left atrial hypertension
• Onset of symptoms within 6 hours of transfusion
• No preexisting ALI before transfusion
	Possible TRALI:
	• New ALI
	• Onset of symptoms within 6 hours of transfusion
	• No preexisting ALI before transfusion
		• New ALI
		• Onset of symptoms within 6 hours of transfusion
		• No preexisting ALI before transfusion
		• Confirmation through assessment of patient's clinical course:
		  – If the new ALI is mechanistically related to the transfusion or both the transfusion and the alternative risk factor, the reaction is TRALI.
		  – If the new ALI is not mechanistically related to the transfusion, the reaction is not TRALI.

*Adapted from Toy et al[7] and Kleinman et al,[8] and reprinted from Kopko and Popovsky.[4]

TRALI = transfusion-related acute lung injury; ALI = acute lung injury; PaO_2 = partial pressure of oxygen in arterial blood; FiO_2 = inspired oxygen concentration; sat = saturated; NHLBI = National Heart, Lung, and Blood Institute.

fines this condition as possible TRALI, whereas the NHLBI defines it as TRALI if the clinical time course suggests that the other risk factors for ALI are unlikely causes.

Clinical Presentation and Complications

TRALI is indistinguishable from ALI secondary to other causes and is often life-threatening. Patients typically present with dyspnea or cyanosis. If the patient is intubated, he or she may present with pink, frothy secretions in the endotracheal tube, or an increase in required inspired oxygen, or both. The symptoms include severe bilateral pulmonary edema and severe hypoxemia (arterial oxygen tensions of 30 to 50 mm Hg are frequent), tachycardia, fever (1 to 2 C increase), and hypertension or hypotension.[4,5,7,9]

Although it may first be confined to the lower lung fields, the edema may progress to involve the entire lung over several hours. Roentgenograms classically demonstrate "whiteout" by interstitial and alveolar infiltrates in severe cases,[4,5] but, in the first few hours, a patchy pattern may be observed. For patients who are in the decubitus position in the operating room, the edema may first manifest itself in dependent areas of the lung. The chest radiographs in TRALI are indistinguishable from other causes of ALI and are difficult to distinguish from cardiogenic pulmonary edema.

The hypotension that is observed is typically mild to moderate (15 to 30 mm Hg decrease from the pretransfusion level). When it occurs, the hypotension is usually unresponsive to fluid administration. The administration of diuretics to the normotensive or hypertensive TRALI patient may induce hypotension. In one report, acute respiratory distress (76%), hypotension (15%), and hypertension (15%) were the most frequent presenting symptoms that led to the diagnosis of TRALI.[10]

All of these symptoms arise in the setting of a recent transfusion of plasma-containing blood components—always within 1 to 6 hours—and, in 90% of cases, within 1 to 2 hours.[4] In contrast to cardiogenic pulmonary edema or volume (circulatory) overload, patients with TRALI have normal or decreased central venous pressure and normal or low pulmonary wedge pressure.[4]

Unlike ALI, with its high morbidity and mortality (30% to 50%), 80% of patients with TRALI improve both clinically and physiologically within 48 to 96 hours of the original insult, provided there is prompt and vigorous respiratory support.[4,5,8,10] In many ALI patients, the lung injury is irreversible, whereas in TRALI patients the pulmonary lesion is typically transient. The arterial PaO_2 levels return to their pretransfusion levels and chest radiographs document the rapid clearing of the edema fluid. In one of the largest studies of this syndrome, 100% of 36 patients required oxygen support, and 72% required short-term mechanical ventilation.[4,5] One subset of patients, however, had a more prolonged course. In about one-fifth of these cases, pulmonary infiltrates persisted for at least 7 days, but even those patients showed no evidence of having permanent sequelae.

In addition to the clinical symptoms, it is now appreciated that TRALI may be associated with acute transient leukopenia. Several reports[11-15] of transient neutropenia, leukopenia, or both are associated with TRALI. The duration of the leukopenia ranges from less than 2 hours[11,12] to approximately 16 hours. Because of this association, a complete blood count with white blood cell differential should be considered as an early part of the investigation of possible cases of TRALI.

When a case of TRALI is recognized, other co-components from the same donation as the implicated unit should be quarantined by the blood bank. Regarding the workup and management of implicated donors, policies differ between institutions (see Chapter 4).

In comparison to other immediate transfusion reactions, TRALI is more severe. Only ABO-hemolytic transfusion reactions have a comparable mortality rate.[16] The fatality rate in TRALI is reported to be 5% to 24%,[10] with the most widely cited figures being 5% to 10%.[5,7] TRALI is the leading cause of transfusion-associated death in the United States.[4,7] In the period from 2001 to 2003, it accounted for 16% of transfusion-related fatalities reported to the Food and Drug Administration (FDA). By 2005, TRALI was responsible for 36.6% of the reported fatalities; in 2006, it accounted for 50.7% of the fatalities.[17]

Mild TRALI

Milder forms of TRALI almost certainly exist that do not meet the consensus definition. Davis et al[18] identified 3 cases that presented with chills, dyspnea, modest temperature increases, and mildly decreased oxygen saturation. In each instance, a blood component containing an HLA antibody reactive with a cognate antigen was identified. Palfi and Holthius[19] found that the majority of cases of TRALI reported through a hemovigilance system in southern Sweden were considered mild and were characterized by impairment of lung function with fever, cyanosis, or tachycardia.

Incidence

The incidence of TRALI is unknown—for multiple reasons: no standard definition before 2004; lack of reliable denominator data on the annual number of components transfused; active case investigation vs passive surveillance; and underrecognition, underreporting, and confusion with other clinical entities, notably transfusion-associated circulatory overload (TACO).[4,8] These factors account for the widely disparate figures that have been reported. From the United States, two frequently cited studies found incidences of 1 in 1300 and 1 in 5000 plasma-containing transfusions, respectively.[5,20] The 1 in 5000 figure is from the Mayo Clinic, where nurses specially trained in transfusion practice and complications are responsible for transfusions outside the operating room, thus providing a degree of vigilance rarely found elsewhere. A prospective study with active electronic surveillance of arterial blood gases of patients after transfusion at two large, academic medical centers found that TRALI occurred in 1 per 3138 units transfused and in 1 per 473 patients transfused before the implementation of any TRALI risk-reduction strategy.[21] In a single-hospital report from the United Kingdom that addressed Fresh Frozen Plasma (FFP) transfusions, the incidence was 1 per 7900 units.[22] The most frequently implicated blood components are FFP, Whole Blood (WB), Red Blood Cells (RBCs), Pooled Platelets, and Apheresis Platelets. Several hemovigilance programs have found that incidence varies widely by component. In 2005 in Quebec, TRALI was diagnosed in 1 per 15,924 FFP units, 1 per 47,484 RBC units, 1 per 40,452 Pooled Platelet units, and 1 per 48,996 Apheresis Platelet units transfused.[23] Lower rates of occurrence have been reported in the United Kingdom[24] and France.[25] Whether those differences by component types reflect the plasma volume, some intrinsic factors, or the type of surveillance is unknown.

A recent nested control study of consecutive intensive care unit patients who did not require respiratory support before transfusion identified TRALI in 1 per 534 transfusions.[26] This study suggests that, in some clinical settings, TRALI is common. Such a view is supported by a look-back study of 50 patients who received plasma components from a donor who was known to have a strong human neutrophil antigen-3a antibody and who was linked to a TRALI fatality in which seven mild or moderate reactions were identified.[27] Of the severe reactions, only two were reported to the transfusion service in the hospital. Repeat reactions in the same patient were also identified. This study suggests that TRALI is both underrecognized and underreported.

Risk Factors

TRALI is evenly distributed among males and females. It has been identified in all age groups, from children to elderly patients.[4,28] A French study found that, of 161 cases, 60 patients

(37%) were 60 years of age or older.[25] A nested case-control study of 46 TRALI patients that was compared with 225 control patients who had received transfusions identified hematologic malignancy and cardiac disease as risk factors for developing TRALI.[20] FDA reports of transfusion-associated deaths indicate an association with cardiovascular surgery, active infection, and hematologic disease.[29] Others have made an association with massive transfusion, thrombotic thrombocytopenic purpura, and surgical procedures.[30] Gajic et al[26] reported that patients in the intensive care unit with ALI were more likely to have sepsis and a history of chronic alcohol abuse.

Differential Diagnosis

Anaphylactic Transfusion Reactions

Respiratory distress and cyanosis related to bronchospasm and laryngeal edema, not pulmonary edema, are the dominant symptoms of an anaphylactic transfusion reaction. Wheezing, chest tightness, and substernal chest pain may be present.[31] Erythema and urticaria are prominent and typically involve confluent areas of the trunk, face, and neck. Hypotension is usually severe and frequently occurs within seconds to minutes after the initiation of transfusion of a plasma-containing blood component or a plasma derivative (with as little as a few milliliters). Fever is not a manifestation of anaphylactic reactions. The frequency of severe reactions is 1 per 20,000 to 1 per 47,000 units transfused.[32,33]

Transfusion-Associated Sepsis

Fever, hypotension, and vascular collapse are prominent features of a reaction related to bacterial contamination of a blood component.[34] Acute transient leukopenia and ALI can also occur. The onset of symptoms is within hours of transfusion of a cellular or plasma-containing blood component. Immediate symptoms are associated with endotoxin from gram-negative bacteria; delayed symptoms, with gram-positive bacteria. Although platelet concentrates or Apheresis Platelets are the most frequently implicated components, RBCs may be involved.[35] A clear diagnosis is made by culturing the same organism with the same antibiotic sensitivities both from the blood product bag and from the patient's peripheral blood.

Circulatory Overload

For patients with diminished cardiac reserve, rapid infusion or large-volume blood component infusion is a precipitating cause of acute pulmonary edema secondary to circulatory overload. Within several hours of transfusion, the patient may develop any or all of the following: dyspnea, orthopnea, cyanosis, tachycardia, pedal edema, or increased blood pressure.[36] Auscultation reveals the presence of rales. Adults older than 60 and infants are especially susceptible to fluid overload. In some vulnerable individuals, 1 to 2 units of blood components are sufficient to trigger TACO. In the intensive care setting, an incidence of 1 in 356 components transfused was reported.[26] In two studies of orthopedic surgical patients, 1% to 8% of patients developed TACO in the immediate postoperative period.[36-38] Because brain natriuretic peptide is elevated in TACO, a test for the peptide may help distinguish TACO from TRALI.[39]

Summary

TRALI is an important clinical diagnosis because of its severe morbidity and high mortality. It is the most frequent cause of death from transfusion therapy and is associated with any plasma-containing blood component. TRALI is both underrecognized and underreported. The incidence rates most frequently cited are 1 per 1300 and 1 per 5000, but widely divergent rates have been reported. Individuals older than 60 years, patients with cardiovascular disease or hematologic malignancy, or those in the intensive care unit setting may be at increased risk for the syndrome. Other risk factors may emerge. A consensus definition, based on clinical data, is being used. Finally, the clinical diagnosis of TRALI can be challenging because TACO, other causes of ALI, and other respiratory complications of transfusion must be considered.

References

1. Carilli AD, Ramanamurty MV, Chang YS, et al. Noncardiogenic pulmonary edema following blood transfusion. Chest 1978;74:310-12.
2. Kernoff PB, Durrant IJ, Rizza CR, Wright FW. Severe allergic pulmonary oedema after plasma transfusion. Br J Haematol 1972;23:777-81.
3. Barnard RD. Indiscriminate transfusions: A critique of case reports illustrating hypersensitivity reactions. N Y State J Med 1951;51:2399-401.
4. Kopko PM, Popovsky MA. Transfusion-related acute lung injury. In: Popovsky MA, ed. Transfusion reactions. 3rd ed. Bethesda, MD: AABB Press, 2007:207-8.
5. Popovsky MA, Moore SB. Diagnostic and pathogenetic considerations in transfusion-related acute lung injury. Transfusion 1985;25:573-7.
6. Bernard GR, Artigas A, Brigham KL, et al. The American-European Consensus Conference on ARDS. Definitions, mechanisms, relevant outcomes, and clinical trial coordination. Am J Respir Crit Care Med 1994;149:818-24.
7. Toy P, Popovsky MA, Abraham E, et al. Transfusion-related acute lung injury: Definition and review. Crit Care Med 2005;33:721-6.
8. Kleinman S, Caulfield T, Chan P, et al. Toward an understanding of transfusion-related acute lung injury: Statement of a consensus panel. Transfusion 2004; 44:1774-89.
9. Popovsky MA, Chaplin HC Jr, Moore SB. Transfusion-related acute lung injury: A neglected, serious complication of hemotherapy. Transfusion 1992;32:589-92.
10. Popovsky MA, Haley NR. Further characterization of transfusion-related acute lung injury: Demographics, clinical and laboratory features, and morbidity. Immunohematology 2000;16:157-9.
11. Leger R, Palm S, Wulf H, et al. Transfusion-related acute lung injury caused by fresh frozen plasma containing anti-NB1. Anesthesiology 1999;91:1529-32.
12. Nakagawa M, Toy P. Acute and transient decrease in neutrophil count in transfusion-related acute lung injury: Cases at one hospital. Transfusion 2004;44: 1689-94.

13. Yomtovian R, Kline W, Press C, et al. Severe pulmonary hypersensitivity associated with passive transfusion of a neutrophil-specific antibody. Lancet 1984;1: 244-6.

14. Ausley MB Jr. Fatal transfusion reactions caused by donor antibodies to recipient leukocytes. Am J Forensic Med Pathol 1987;4:287-90.

15. Looney MR, Gropper MA, Matthay MA. Transfusion-related acute lung injury (TRALI): A review. Chest 2004;126:249-58.

16. Davenport RD. Hemolytic transfusion reactions. In: Popovsky MA, ed. Transfusion reactions. 3rd ed. Bethesda, MD: AABB Press, 2007:1-55.

17. Holness L. Presentation on discussion of transfusion-related acute lung injury from the Blood Products Advisory Committee meeting of April 27, 2007. Meeting of the Advisory Committee on Blood Product Safety and Availability, Department of Health and Human Services, Rockville, MD, May 10, 2007.

18. Davis A, Makar R, Stowell C, Dzik S. Pathophysiology of TRALI: Are there lessons from mild cases not meeting the current consensus definitions? (abstract). Transfusion 2007;47(Suppl 3S):105A.

19. Palfi P, Holthius N. Does mild TRALI exist? Analysis of one-year transfusion complications from south Sweden (abstract). Vox Sang 2004;87(Suppl 3):5.

20. Silliman CC, Boshkov LK, Mehdizadehkashi Z, et al. Transfusion-related acute lung injury: Epidemiology and a prospective analysis of etiologic factors. Blood 2003;101:454-62.

21. Toy P, Gajic O, Gropper M. Prospective assessment of the incidence of TRALI (abstract). Transfusion 2007;47(Suppl 3S):7A.

22. Wallis JP, Lubenko A, Wells AW, Chapman CE. Single hospital experience of TRALI. Transfusion 2003;43:1053-9.

23. Robillard P, Hyson C, McCombie N. TRALI, possible TRALI, and respiratory complications of transfusion reported to the Canadian Transfusion Transmitted Injuries Surveillance system (abstract). Transfusion 2007;47(Suppl 3S):5-6A.

24. Goldman M, Webert KE, Arnold DM, et al. Proceedings of a Consensus Conference: Towards an understanding of TRALI. Transfus Med Rev 2005;19:2-31.

25. Renaudier P, Mai MV, Ounnouhghhene N, et al. Epidemiology of transfusion-related acute lung injury in e-FIT, the French Hemovigilance Network (abstract). Transfusion 2007;47(Suppl 3S):7A.

26. Gajic O, Rana R, Winters J, et al. Transfusion-related acute lung injury in the critically ill: Prospective nested-control study. Am J Respir Crit Care Med 2007; 176:1-6.

27. Kopko PM, Marshall CS, Mackenzie MR, et al. Transfusion-related acute lung injury: Report of a clinical look-back case. JAMA 2002;287:1968-71.

28. Church GD, Price C, Sanchez R, Looney MR. Transfusion-related acute lung injury in the paediatric patient: Two case reports and a review of the literature. Transfus Med, 2006;16:343-8.

29. Holness L, Knippen MA, Simmons L, Lachenbruch PA. Fatalities caused by TRALI. Transfus Med Rev 2004;18:184-8.

30. Bux J, Sachs UJ. The pathogenesis of transfusion-related acute lung injury. Br J Haematol 2007;136:788-9.

31. Vamvakas EC. Allergic and anaphylactic reactions. In: Popovsky MA, ed. Transfusion reactions. 3rd ed. Bethesda, MD: AABB Press, 2007:105-56.

32. Bjerrum OJ, Jersild C. Class-specific anti-IgA associated with severe anaphylactic transfusion reactions in a patient with pernicious anemia. Vox Sang 1971; 21:411-24.

33. Pineda AA, Taswell HF. Transfusion reactions associated with anti-IgA antibodies: Report of four cases and review of the literature. Transfusion 1975;15:10-15.

34. Ramírez-Arcos S, Goldman M, Blajchman MA. Bacterial contamination. In: Popovsky MA, ed. Transfusion reactions. 3rd ed. Bethesda, MD: AABB Press, 2007:163-206.

35. Blajchman MA, Beckers EAM, Dickmeiss E, et al. Bacterial detection of platelets: Current problems and possible resolutions. Transfus Med Rev 2005;19: 259-72.

36. Popovsky M. Circulatory overload. In: Popovsky MA, ed. Transfusion reactions. 3rd ed. Bethesda, MD: AABB Press, 2007:331-40.

37. Popovsky M, Audet AM, Andrzewski C Jr. Transfusion-associated circulatory overload in orthopedic surgery patients: A multi-institutional study. Immunohematology 1996;12:87-9.

38. Bierbaum BE, Callaghan JJ, Galante JO. An analysis of blood management in patients having a total knee or hip arthroplasty. J Bone Joint Surg Am 1999; 81:2-10.

39. Zhou L, Giacherion D, Cooling L, Davenport RD. Use of B-natriuretic peptide as a diagnostic marker in the differential diagnosis of transfusion-associated circulatory overload. Transfusion 2005;45:1056-63.

In: Kleinman S, Popovsky MA, eds.
TRALI: Mechanisms, Management, and Prevention
Bethesda, MD: AABB Press, 2008

2

Transfusion and Acute Lung Injury in the Critically Ill

HASRAT KHAN, MD;
RODRIGO CARTIN-CEBA, MD; AND
OGNJEN GAJIC, MD, MSc

TRANSFUSIONS ARE REGULARLY USED IN THE care of the critically ill. With regular testing of viral pathogens in donated blood leading to a marked decrease in transmission of infectious disease, transfusion-related acute lung injury (TRALI) has emerged as the most common serious complication of blood transfusion.[1,2] Although reported TRALI has become the most impor-

Hasrat Khan, MD, Intensivist, Department of Critical Care Services, MeritCare Medical Center, Fargo, North Dakota; Rodrigo Cartin-Ceba, MD, Critical Care Fellow, Division of Pulmonary and Critical Care Medicine, Mayo Clinic, Rochester, Minnesota; and Ognjen Gajic, MD, MSc, Senior Associate Consultant and Associate Professor of Medicine, Division of Pulmonary and Critical Care Medicine, Mayo Clinic, Rochester, Minnesota

tant cause of transfusion-related mortality, most transfusion specialists, intensivists, anesthesiologists, and other physicians consider it a rare disorder.[3] Distinct pathophysiologic mechanisms have been supported by both animal models and clinical studies.[4-9] Large amounts of blood components are transfused to critically ill surgical or medical patients with acute bleeding, up to 40% of whom develop acute lung injury (ALI).[2] Although ALI and its more severe form—acute respiratory distress syndrome (ARDS)—are often attributed to an underlying reason for transfusion (shock), emerging evidence from randomized[10,11] and observational[12-22] studies suggests not only that transfusion itself is an important etiologic factor but also that mechanisms implicated in the development of TRALI play an important role, perhaps as co-factors, in many patients who develop ALI/ARDS temporally related to transfusion.[4,15,23,24] Because of the complexity of the clinical evaluation of critically ill patients,[25] these mechanisms are neither reported to nor investigated by the blood bank, leading to widespread underrecognition.[4,15]

To enhance the reproductivity of clinical studies of TRALI, a recent consensus conference[26] suggested the use of two specific terms to characterize ALI/ARDS that develops in temporal proximity to transfusion: "TRALI" (if transfusion is the only plausible etiologic factor) and "possible TRALI" (in the presence of other ALI/ARDS risk factors: sepsis, aspiration, trauma). However, in recent studies of transfused critically ill patients in which the investigators used recommended standard definitions, specific transfusion factors appeared to be independently linked to the development of ALI/ARDS regardless of the presence or absence of other ALI/ARDS risk factors.[15,24] Analogous to ischemic heart disease where multiple etiologic factors (eg, hypertension, hypercholesterolemia, smoking) interact to increase the probability of a heart attack, multiple factors (aspiration, trauma, shock, mechanical ventilation, *and* transfusion) are likely to be involved in the development and expression of ALI/ARDS. In critically ill patients, transfusion factors clearly contribute to the risk of ALI/ARDS after blood transfusions; furthermore, these factors may be even more important prevention targets in patients who have multiple additional ALI/ARDS risk factors than in those who do not.[12,24]

However, TRALI remains underrecognized by clinicians, including intensivists, because they lack awareness of the condition and the presence of multiple confounding factors such as sepsis, aspiration, pneumonia, and trauma that could explain ALI/ARDS. With increasing health-care costs and the continuous emphasis on improvement in patient care, it is of paramount importance both to define this transfusion-related phenomenon better and to design effective strategies for its prevention.

Epidemiology

In a critique of case reports showing "hypersensitivity reactions," Barnard[27] in 1951 had reported features that could constitute the syndrome of TRALI. However, TRALI as a clinical entity was first recognized by Popovsky et al in 1983[28] and again by Popovsky and Moore in 1985.[5] Since then, it has emerged as one of the most serious complications of blood transfusion.[4,5,28,29]

The incidence of TRALI has varied according to case definitions and methods of surveillance and data collection on components transfused. Most literature generally refers to a range of anywhere between one case per 1200 transfusions in observational studies to one per 500,000 transfusions in passive surveillance systems.[26] This latter rate is felt to be a gross underestimate because the majority of cases are typically neither recognized nor reported. For example, Kopko et al[4] did a retrospective review of 36 patient charts on the recommendation of the US Food and Drug Administration (FDA) in a look-back investigation of transfusion-related fatalities. Of the 36 patients who were transfused Fresh Frozen Plasma (FFP) from one particular donor (a 54-year-old multiparous female), 13 (36%) had transfusion reactions. Of the eight severe reactions involving ALI/ARDS, TRALI was considered in the differential diagnosis of only two. It is reasonable to suspect that all eight patients had TRALI.

Until recently,[26] there was no uniform definition of TRALI. Various studies used different definitions, which presumably either underdiagnosed or overdiagnosed TRALI. Most studies have excluded patients with any other known cause of ALI, such as sepsis, pneumonia, aspiration, and trauma. Hence, patients who developed ALI in these settings were not considered to have developed TRALI.[2,26] Transfusion in these settings, however, could have either a primary or a contributory role in the development of ALI (multiple hit hypothesis).

Massive Transfusion as a Risk Factor for ALI

In four observational studies,[16,17,30,31] both the risk factor (multiple transfusions) and the outcome (ALI/ARDS) were studied in a defined patient population free of ALI/ARDS at study inception (Table 2-1).[32]

Pepe et al[30] studied 136 patients during an 18-month period in the late 1970s and early 1980s at Harborview Medical Center in Seattle, Washington. This group used the term "multiple emergency transfusions" to define those patients who received >10 units of whole blood or Red Blood Cells (RBCs) within 12 hours. The primary outcome studied was ARDS defined as 1) partial pressure of oxygen in arterial blood (PaO_2) <75 torr with inspired oxygen concentration (FiO_2) of 0.5, 2) new diffuse bilateral infiltrates (all lung fields involved) on a chest roentgenogram, 3) pulmonary artery wedge pressure <18 mm Hg, and 4) no other explanation for the above findings.

Of the 136 patients with one of eight identified predispositions (sepsis syndrome, aspiration of gastric contents, pulmonary contusion, multiple emergency transfusions, multiple major fractures, near-drowning, pancreatitis, and prolonged hypotension), 42 met the multiple emergency transfusions criteria either alone or in combination with one of the other predispositions. Of the 42 patients, 19 (45%) developed ARDS, yielding an odds ratio of 2.05 [95% confidence interval (CI), 0.96-4.36].

Table 2-1. Massive Transfusion as a Risk Factor for ALI

Study	Design	Study Patients	Multiple Transfusion Definition	ALI/ARDS Definition	Odds Ratio	95% CI
Pepe et al[30]	Prospective, observational	136	>10 units whole blood or RBCs in 12 hours	• PaO_2 <75 torr with FiO_2 ≥0.5 • New diffuse bilateral infiltrates • Pulmonary artery wedge pressure <18 mm Hg	2.05	0.96-4.36
Hudson et al[31]	Prospective, observational	695	≥15 units in 24 hours	• PaO_2/FiO_2 ≤150 or PaO_2/FiO_2 ≤200 on positive end-expiratory pressure • Diffuse infiltrates involving all lung quadrants • Pulmonary artery wedge pressure <18 mm Hg or no clinical evidence of congestive heart failure	2.24	1.47-3.41

(Continued)

Table 2-1. Massive Transfusion as a Risk Factor for ALI (Continued)

Study	Design	Study Patients	Multiple Transfusion Definition	ALI/ARDS Definition	Odds Ratio	95% CI
Gong et al[16]	Prospective, observational	189	≥8 units RBCs in 24 hours	• Intubated on positive ventilation • $PaO_2/FiO_2 \leq 200$ mm Hg • Otherwise unexplained bilateral infiltrates • Pulmonary arterial occlusion pressure ≤18 mm Hg or no clinical evidence of left atrial hypertension	0.89*	0.39-2.05
Silverboard et al[17]	Prospective, observational	102	Not defined; presumed >10 units RBCs	Standard AECC definition	14.4	3.2-78.7

*Many "control" patients received submassive transfusion; see Table 2-2.
ALI = acute lung injury; ARDS = acute respiratory distress syndrome; CI = confidence interval; RBCs = Red Blood Cells; PaO_2/FiO_2 = partial pressure of oxygen in arterial blood/inspired oxygen concentration; AECC = American-European Consensus Conference. (Adapted from Belsher et al[32] with permission from Springer Science and Business Media.)

Hudson et al,[31] also from Harborview Medical Center, studied 695 patients who presented to the 38-bed intensive care unit (ICU) from 1983 through 1985. This group also used the term multiple emergency transfusions but this time defined it to include those patients who received ≥15 units of blood within 24 hours. The primary outcome studied was ARDS defined as 1) $PaO_2/FiO_2 \leq 150$ or $PaO_2/FiO_2 \leq 200$ on positive end-expiratory pressure (PEEP), 2) diffuse infiltrates that involved all lung quadrants on a chest roentgenogram, 3) pulmonary artery wedge pressure <18 mm Hg (if available) or no clinical evidence of congestive heart failure, and 4) no other explanation for the above findings.

Of the 695 patients with one of eight identified predispositions (sepsis syndrome, aspiration, drug overdose, near-drowning, pulmonary contusion, multiple transfusions, multiple fractures, and head trauma), 115 met the multiple emergency transfusions criteria either alone or in combination with one of the other predispositions. Of the 115, 46 (40%) developed ARDS, yielding an odds ratio of 2.24 (95% CI, 1.47-3.41).

Gong et al[33] studied 189 patients admitted to the neurological, cardiac, medical, and surgical ICUs of Massachusetts General Hospital between September 1999 and March 2001. This group used the term "multiple transfusions" to define those patients who received ≥8 units of RBCs within 24 hours. The primary outcome studied was again ARDS defined as 1) the patient intubated on positive pressure ventilation; 2) PaO_2/FiO_2 ≤200 mm Hg; 3) bilateral infiltrates seen on chest radiographs not fully explained by masses, effusions, or collapse; and 4) pulmonary arterial occlusion pressure ≤18 mm Hg or no clinical evidence of left atrial hypertension.

Of the 189 patients with one of five identified predispositions (sepsis, septic shock, trauma, multiple transfusions, and aspiration), 28 met the multiple transfusions criteria either alone or in combination with one of the other predispositions. Of the 28 patients, 10 (36%) developed ARDS.

In a prospective cohort study of 102 trauma patients who were stratified in three groups according to the number of units of RBCs transfused (group 1 = 0 to 5 units, group 2 = 6 to 10 units, and group 3 = more than 10 units), Silverboard et al[17] found an increased risk for developing ARDS in those receiving >10 units of RBCs as compared to those receiving 0 to 5 units (odds ratio or OR, 14.1; 95% CI, 3.2 to 78.7). This study also demonstrated a dose-response relationship between the number of units transfused and the risk of developing ARDS in both blunt and penetrating trauma patients. When blunt trauma patients were stratified on the basis of those receiving ≤5 units vs >5 units of RBCs, the risk of developing ARDS rose sharply from 27% to 70% (p = 0.001). When penetrating trauma patients were stratified on the basis of those receiving ≤10 units vs >10 units, the risk of developing ARDS again rose sharply from 6% to 46% (p = 0.002).

It is important to realize that critically ill patients who undergo massive RBC transfusion are universally exposed to non-RBC components, including FFP and platelets. In a recent study in medical critical care patients, 75% of patients who received >10 units of RBCs also received FFP or platelets, and the transfusion of non-RBC components was a significant predictor of ALI development.[22]

Although demonstration of a dose-response relationship is an important feature in establishing causality, the following preclude comparisons between studies and limit the ability to determine causal relationships: the absence of proper accounting for confounding factors, different study populations, lack of consensus on a uniform definition of TRALI when most of the previously mentioned studies were performed, and differences in time periods and transfusion exposures.

Submassive Transfusion as a Risk Factor for ALI

Historically, submassive (any) transfusion has not been considered a risk factor for ALI/ARDS. However, evidence to the contrary is slowly growing (see Table 2-2). The strongest evidence for a causal relationship between transfusion and the development of ALI/ARDS comes from the landmark study of the Ca-

Table 2-2. Submassive Transfusion as a Risk Factor for ALI

Study	Design	Study Patients	Transfusion Definition	ALI/ARDS Definition	Odds Ratio	95% CI
Hébert et al[11]	Prospective, interventional	418 restrictive 420 liberal	Any number of units*	Not specified	0.64 restrictive 1.5 liberal	0.40-1.03 0.97-2.49
Gajic et al[20]	Retrospective, observational	181	Any number of units	Standard AECC definition	2.28	1.16-4.59
Gong et al[16]	Prospective, observational	688	Any number of units	Standard AECC definition	2.19	1.42-3.36
Khan et al[22]	Retrospective, observational	841	Any number of units	Standard AECC definition	2.14	1.24-3.75
Croce et al[34]	Retrospective, observational	5260	Any number of units	$PaO_2/FiO_2 <200$ mm Hg, PPV, bilateral infiltrate on CXR No evidence of CHF, and Ppk >50 cm H_2O	3.42 (p <0.001)	—

(Continued)

Table 2-2. Submassive Transfusion as a Risk Factor for ALI (Continued)

Study	Design	Study Patients	Transfusion Definition	ALI/ARDS Definition	Odds Ratio	95% CI
Zilberberg et al[18]	Prospective, observational	4892	Any number of units	PaO$_2$/FiO$_2$ <200 mm Hg, bilateral infiltrate on CXR, pulmonary artery occlusion pressure ≤18 mm Hg when measured, or no clinical evidence of left atrial hypertension	2.74	2.09-3.49

*All patients in the liberal group and 70% of patients in the restrictive group were transfused.

ALI = acute lung injury; ARDS = acute respiratory distress syndrome; CI = confidence interval; AECC = American-European Consensus Conference; PaO$_2$/FiO$_2$ = partial pressure of oxygen in arterial blood/inspired oxygen concentration; PPV = positive pressure ventilation; CXR = chest x-ray; CHF = congestive heart failure; Ppk = peak airway pressure. (Adapted from Belsher et al[32] with permission from Springer Science and Business Media.)

nadian Critical Care Trials Group.[11] In this study, 838 critically ill patients who were admitted to ICUs for more than 24 hours were randomized to either a liberal strategy (hemoglobin threshold for transfusion of 10 g/dL) or a restrictive strategy (hemoglobin threshold for transfusion of 7 g/dL). On average, the restrictive group received 2.6 units, whereas the liberal group received 5.6 units of blood. ALI/ARDS developed in ≈11% of patients in the liberal group and ≈8% of patients in the restrictive group. The odds ratio for the development of ALI/ARDS was 1.56 (95% CI, 0.97-2.49) in patients assigned to the liberal as opposed to the restrictive transfusion group. More recently, Boffard et al[10] demonstrated a significant decrease in the incidence of ALI/ARDS in massively transfused blunt trauma patients who were randomized to recombinant Factor VII and who received smaller quantities of FFP.

Multiple observational studies suggested that transfusion factors may play a significant role in the development of ALI.[12-22] In a retrospective cohort of 332 critically ill patients mechanically ventilated for 48 hours or longer, 180 of whom were transfused, 80 subsequently developed ALI/ARDS.[20] Having received a transfusion of one or more units (ie, any transfusion) and having large initial tidal volumes were identified as the most important risk factors for the development of ALI/ARDS. In a multivariate analysis, the odds ratio for development of ALI/ARDS in the transfused patients was 2.97 (95% CI, 1.56-5.9). In a more recent study from the same institution, any transfusion was once again shown to be independently associated with development of ALI/ARDS (OR = 2.14; 95% CI, 1.24-3.75).[22] In terms of individual blood products, any platelet and FFP transfusion had a stronger independent association with the development of ALI/ARDS than did an RBC transfusion.[14,22] Another study observed the occurrence of ALI and postprocedural bleeding in patients with coagulopathy but without active bleeding who either received or did not receive prophylactic FFP. Although there was no difference in bleeding complications, patients exposed to prophylactic FFP were more likely to develop ALI.[19] Therefore, receipt of an FFP transfusion in a majority of the case series and case reports of TRALI[2,3] is being substantiated in the critically ill patient population.

Similar to FFP transfusion, platelet transfusion was also found to have a stronger independent association with the development of ALI/ARDS than did RBC transfusion.[22] In another study of platelet transfusion practice in the ICU, 90 of the 117 patients who were included in the study received platelet transfusion. Of the 90 patients who received platelet transfusion, 6 developed transfusion complications; of the 6, 2 were diagnosed as having TRALI.[35]

In an observational prospective study by Gong et al,[16] 688 patients admitted to Massachusetts General Hospital with one of four risk factors for ALI/ARDS (sepsis, trauma, aspiration, or multiple transfusions) were studied for a genetic predisposition to ALI/ARDS. The authors observed that any amount of transfusion was independently associated with increased odds of developing ALI/ARDS (OR = 2.19; 95% CI, 1.42-3.36). In particular, those transfused with ≤3 units had increasing rates of ALI/ARDS. However, the results of this study may not be applicable to all ICU patients because the authors studied only those with known risk factors for ALI/ARDS.

Croce et al, in a retrospective review[34] of 5260 patients who were admitted to a trauma ICU with an Injury Severity Score (ISS) <25, demonstrated a much higher risk of ALI/ARDS in those who were transfused (2.8%) when compared to those who were not transfused (0.2%). The calculated relative risk increase for ALI/ARDS in those who received any transfusion was approximately 92.9%. In their multivariate logistics regression analysis, transfusion was independently associated with the development of ALI/ARDS (OR = 3.42; p <0.001). Similar findings were obtained in a recent multicenter cohort study by Zilberberg et al.[18] A causal relationship between transfusion and ALI/ARDS can be suggested but cannot be confirmed by these observational studies.

Several recent studies explored the relationship between specific transfusion factors such as donor gender, parity, and product storage time and the development of ALI/ARDS in critically ill patients. In a retrospective study by Rana et al,[23] the total amount of plasma and the amount of female plasma—but not the storage age of RBCs or the percentage of leukocyte reduction—were associated with development of clinical TRALI in critically ill patients. A subsequent prospective study confirmed and expanded these findings.[15] Mayo Clinic researchers investigated the incidence, risk factors, and outcome of ALI that develops within 6 hours after transfusion in patients admitted to the medical ICU. Of 901 patients, 74 (8%) developed ALI within 6 hours of transfusion. Patients with sepsis, liver disease, and a history of chronic alcohol abuse were more likely than other patients to develop ALI, as were patients who received plasma-rich blood components, components from female donors, and larger volumes of plasma from female donors. Donors to patients who subsequently developed ALI had a higher number of pregnancies and tested positive for leukocyte antibodies more often than did donors to patients who did not develop ALI. Interleukin-8 (IL-8) concentrations and the storage age of red cell components did not differ between patients who developed ALI and matched controls, but the concentration of lysophosphatidylcholine (lyso-PC) was significantly higher in components given to ALI case subjects than to control subjects. Hospital mortality was significantly higher in patients who developed ALI (41%) than in matched controls (23%).

Perhaps the strongest evidence regarding the role of specific donor factors in the development of ALI in critically ill patients comes from a recent United Kingdom (UK) study, in which the investigators observed a significant decrease in the development of ALI in patients undergoing a repair of ruptured abdominal aneurysms after the introduction of predominantly male-donor FFP in the UK.[24]

Pathogenesis of TRALI

In the past, the relationship between transfusion and ALI/ARDS has been thought to be directly attributable to the underlying illness, where transfusion was merely a marker of the severity of the underlying illness. However, several distinct mechanisms have been described to explain the potential direct causal role of transfusion in the development of ALI/ARDS. Two of the leading theories involve the passive transfer of either leukocyte antibodies or biologic response modifiers in a primed susceptible host. Both of these mechanisms have been reproduced in animal models of TRALI (Fig 2-1).[6,7,9] These two pathogenetic mechanisms may not be mutually exclusive, and both seem to require additional predisposing conditions leading to pulmonary endothelial activation.[36] Risk factors such as sep-

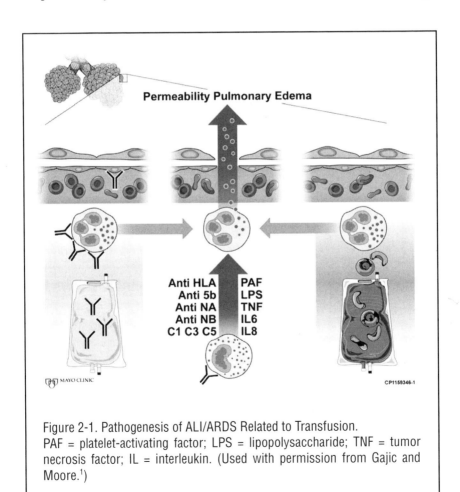

Figure 2-1. Pathogenesis of ALI/ARDS Related to Transfusion.
PAF = platelet-activating factor; LPS = lipopolysaccharide; TNF = tumor necrosis factor; IL = interleukin. (Used with permission from Gajic and Moore.[1])

sis, trauma, pneumonia, or major surgery may serve as the initial priming events ("multiple hit hypothesis").[5,36] In a recent review of pathogenesis of TRALI by Bux and Sachs,[37] the multiple hit hypothesis has been presented as the "threshold model of TRALI" (see Chapter 3).

Passive Transfer of Leukocyte Antibodies

The passive transfer of leukocyte antibodies from multiparous or sensitized donors is the traditional theory of TRALI pathogenesis.[5,29,38] The antibody-mediated increase in pulmonary capillary permeability leads to pulmonary edema and ALI/ARDS. The antibodies in donor blood are thought to be directed against a variety of leukocyte antigens in the host's system, including HLA Class I, HLA Class II (which are expressed on neutrophils and endothelium), and more specific human neutrophil antigens (HNA, expressed only on neutrophils).[37]

During pregnancy, mothers are typically exposed to alloantigens that prime their immune system. The rate of alloimmunization correlates directly with parity as described by Insunza et al[39]: the percentage of female donors with leukocyte antibodies after one, two, or three pregnancies was approximately 9%, 18%, and 23%, respectively. In the original case series of TRALI, Popovsky and Moore[5] found leukocyte antibodies in 85% of the donors whose blood was implicated in the development of TRALI.

The strongest evidence yet for the role of multiparous donors in the pathogenesis of TRALI comes from a recent clinical trial.[38] In a randomized crossover design, 100 patients requiring at least 2 units of FFP were infused with blood from both a nulliparous and a multiparous donor. After receiving the unit of multiparous blood, patients were found to have greater decreases in their PaO_2/FiO_2 ratios and increased levels of circulating tumor necrosis factor alpha (TNF-α).

Bray et al[40] explored the incidence of HLA antibodies in various blood components. They randomly selected 308 units of RBCs, platelets, FFP, and cryoprecipitate. Leukocyte antibodies were found to be present, surprisingly, in 22% of these units. FFP and cryoprecipitate were found to have the highest incidence (29% and 24%, respectively), whereas RBCs had the lowest (12%). In a recent retrospective cohort study of 841 consecutive critically ill patients, Khan et al[22] found a stronger independent association of ALI/ARDS development with transfusion of FFP (OR = 2.48; 95% CI, 1.29-4.74) and platelets (OR = 3.89; 95% CI, 1.36-11.52) than with RBCs (OR = 1.39; 95% CI, 0.79-2.43).

Why does the medical community not see a higher rate of TRALI, given this relatively high incidence of leukocyte antibodies in donor blood? Underrecognition may only partially explain this phenomenon. This mechanism may require specific antigen-antibody pairing between the donor and recipient, as well as achieving a certain concentration threshold of leukocyte antibodies to initiate neutrophil priming and activation, leading to an overwhelming inflammatory response that results in alveolar-capillary membrane damage in a predisposed patient. Accordingly, the amount or concentration of passively transferred antibodies is likely a key determinant of the severity of the reaction.[6] The necessary exact concentration or threshold amount of these antibodies remains to be elucidated.[37] Additionally, preexisting endothelial activation likely serves to potentiate the antigen-antibody reaction.[36]

Biologic Response Modifiers in Stored Cellular Blood Components

Biologic response modifiers such as proinflammatory cytokines (IL-6, IL-8, and TNF-α) and lyso-PCs are known to accumulate during storage of cellular blood components. In animal and ex-vivo models, these mediators trigger an inflammatory cascade, leading to injury of the alveolar-capillary membrane and, consequently, pulmonary edema.[9] The study by Silliman et al[8] demonstrated that the levels of neutrophil priming activity with IL-6 and IL-8 increased with the duration of storage time of the transfused units in the patients who ultimately developed

TRALI. It is believed that the primary culprits in the development of these circulating inflammatory mediators present in stored blood are residual leukocytes. These leukocytes act on erythrocyte membranes causing the release of bioactive lipids, which accumulate in greater concentrations the longer the component is stored. It remains to be seen if universal prestorage leukocyte reduction, currently performed in many countries, will lead to a decreased incidence of TRALI.[26] In an adjusted analysis, the period after universal leukocyte reduction was implemented was not associated with a significant reduction in the incidence of ALI/ARDS.[22] However, this study[22] was not designed to determine the effect of leukocyte reduction on the development of TRALI.

Summary of Pathogenesis

An additional mechanism that may cause or contribute to the development of TRALI is the depletion of nitric oxide in stored components, which may result in pulmonary vasoconstriction and a consequent increase in hydrostatic pressure.[41] This is especially true with multiple transfusions.

Although each of the mechanisms just described seems plausible, it is doubtful that one explains the entire process. To the contrary, it is likely that, in many instances, there is interplay among several mechanisms. In any case, neutrophil priming and activation and endothelial damage seem to be the core components in the pathogenesis of TRALI.[37] A better understanding of the underlying TRALI mechanisms is necessary before it is possible to design effective prevention strategies.

Diagnosis and Differential Diagnosis of TRALI in the ICU

The diagnosis of TRALI is not an easy task, particularly in critically ill patients with acute bleeding, up to 40% of whom develop ALI.[2] Besides those who received transfusion for acute bleeding, critically ill patients are often transfused to correct coagulopathies, to decrease the risk of bleeding during interventional procedures, or are transfused with RBCs to improve oxygen delivery during the early resuscitation of septic shock.[42] Diagnosing TRALI in these situations is problematic because ALI is often attributed to the underlying condition that precipitated the transfusion. Recent literature from randomized[10,11] and observational[1,12,14-17,21,23,43] studies has suggested not only that the transfusion itself is an important etiologic factor but also that mechanisms implicated in the development of TRALI play an important role, perhaps as cofactors, in many patients who develop ALI temporally related to transfusion.[4,22,44,45]

Clinically, TRALI presents with common findings that are also frequently present in other critical care syndromes, including bilateral diffuse crackles, decreased breath sounds, dyspnea, fever, frothy sputum production, cyanosis, tachypnea, and hypotension. Although the latter was initially described in early reports of TRALI,[5,46] it has not been a consistent finding in more recent studies.[8,15] Physiologic abnormalities found in TRALI include acute onset of hypoxemia, with a PaO_2/FiO_2 ratio <300 mm Hg and with decreased pulmonary compliance.[5,8,47] Laboratory findings for TRALI are nonspecific and may include acute transient neutropenia. In addition, radiologic findings are described as diffuse bilateral infiltrates consistent with pulmonary edema.[5] Some of these findings are parts of the 1994 consensus definition on ALI and ARDS,[48] which established the diagnosis of ALI (Table 2-3).

To standardize the definition of TRALI for clinical and research purposes, a consensus conference that was held in Toronto, Canada, during 2004[26,49] defined TRALI as a new episode of ALI that occurs during or within 6 hours of a completed transfusion and that is not temporally related to a competing etiology for ALI. The National Heart, Lung, and Blood Institute's working group on TRALI proposed a very similar definition.[2]

Although the application of a standardized definition can help to differentiate ALI from hydrostatic pulmonary edema,

Table 2-3. Diagnostic Criteria for Acute Lung Injury[48]

Clinical Finding	Criteria
Onset	Acute
Oxygenation	PaO_2/FiO_2 ratio ≤ 300 mm Hg
Chest x-ray	Bilateral infiltrates consistent with pulmonary edema seen on a frontal chest x-ray
Left atrial hypertension	Pulmonary artery wedge pressure ≤ 18 mm Hg or no clinical evidence of left atrial hypertension

PaO_2/FiO_2 = partial pressure of oxygen in arterial blood/inspired oxygen concentration.

distinguishing TRALI from other causes of ALI, such as sepsis, trauma, aspiration, pneumonia, or ventilator-associated lung injury, is all but impossible solely on clinical grounds when one or more of these conditions is present. The differential diagnosis of ALI other than TRALI is beyond the scope of this chapter. Most important, these conditions do not exclude transfusion as an etiologic factor in cases where multiple factors may interact, leading to a full expression of ALI syndrome.

It is important to consider in the differential diagnosis other clinical entities associated with transfusion that can manifest respiratory symptoms similar to TRALI, such as transfusion-associated circulatory overload (TACO), transfusion-associated dyspnea (TAD), and other pulmonary reactions associated with transfusion, including bronchospasm and laryngoedema, that occasionally may accompany allergic transfusion reactions. Moreover, dyspnea may be a prominent feature of acute febrile and hemolytic reactions.

Transfusion-Associated Circulatory Overload

TACO appears to be a relatively common, although underrecognized, complication of blood transfusion.[50] Only a few studies have defined the incidence of TACO, and estimates vary from <1% in hemovigilance reports to 8% in elderly patients after joint replacement surgery.[50,51] In a retrospective study using a custom-designed electronic surveillance system, investigators at the Mayo Clinic recently identified TACO in 25 of 1351 critically ill medical and surgical patients who did not require respiratory support at the onset of transfusion.[52] In a subsequent prospective study in critically ill medical patients, TACO was observed in 69 of 901 patients, suggesting a remarkably high incidence of 8% in this population.[15]

The clinical presentation of TACO is similar to other causes of hydrostatic pulmonary edema. In addition to dyspnea, tachypnea, and jugular venous distension, elevated systolic and diastolic blood pressure and widened pulse pressure are usually present.[50] Although signs of fluid overload are usually present before transfusion, transfusion may precipitate acute hydrostatic pulmonary edema.[50]

Transfusion-Associated Dyspnea

Mild pulmonary reactions that do not meet the consensus conference criteria for TRALI[26] or the diagnostic criteria for TACO frequently occur after blood transfusions.[8,44] In a prospective study in critically ill medical patients, some worsening in respiratory status after the transfusion was observed in more than one-third of the critically ill patients.[44] The European Hemovigilance International Working Group suggested a new term: TAD, which refers to acute respiratory distress without evidence of TRALI, TACO, or allergic reaction. At present, little is understood about this condition, which could conceivably be caused by multiple mechanisms.

Clinical Approach to Differentiation of Acute Pulmonary Transfusion Reactions in the Critically Ill

Bedside clinical information is of paramount importance in order to perform an adequate differential diagnosis of pulmonary transfusion reactions. Table 2-4 lists clinical data that should be abstracted from medical records at the time of the event. The differentiation between ALI (ie, TRALI) and hydrostatic pulmonary edema (TACO) poses a particular challenge because the clinical and radiological manifestations of ALI and hydrostatic pulmonary edema are often similar. The diagnostic differentiation is especially troublesome in critically ill patients with multiple comorbidities so that the cause of edema may be determined only after the fact on the basis of the clinical course and response to therapy. In addition, the two conditions may coexist with about 25% of patients with ALI having a component of hydrostatic pulmonary edema.[44,53] Noninvasive echocardiography and brain natriuretic peptide measurements may aid in the differential diagnosis, and invasive techniques such as right heart catheterization are sometimes helpful. In patients with an endotracheal tube in place, high protein concentration in the edema fluid, if sampled within the first hour of intubation, may help in differentiating ALI from hydrostatic pulmonary edema.

Given the complexity in differential diagnosis of pulmonary transfusion reactions, it is of utmost importance that bedside clinicians and transfusion medicine specialists work together closely in the assessment of patients suspected of having pulmonary transfusion reactions. After collecting appropriate clinical information (Table 2-4) and discussing the case with the clinician, the transfusion medicine specialist should determine the most likely cause of the pulmonary reaction. In the instances where, after thorough review, it appears that the patient has clinical evidence of both ALI and circulatory overload, the case should be classified as ALI, with appropriate implications for prognosis and for donor or component management. A systematic standardized approach to the assessment of pulmonary

Table 2-4. Clinical Information That May Assist in Differential Diagnosis of Pulmonary Transfusion Reactions

Clinical Information	Rationale
History of cardiac dysfunction, sepsis, aspiration, IgA deficiency, or fluid balance before transfusion	• Underlying cardiac dysfunction and positive fluid balance may suggest TACO. • Sepsis and aspiration during the 24 hours before a pulmonary reaction suggest "possible TRALI." • IgA deficiency may suggest an allergic reaction.
Physical examination: fever, systolic and diastolic blood pressure, jugular venous distension, dyspnea, tachypnea, stridor, wheezing, skin changes (urticaria)	• Sudden elevation of blood pressure, jugular venous distension, and wheezing suggest TACO. • Hypotension suggests TRALI. • Stridor, wheezing, and urticaria suggest an allergic reaction. • Fever suggests a febrile reaction or sepsis/bacterial contamination.
Chest x-ray	• The x-ray establishes the presence of bilateral infiltrates/pulmonary edema (TACO or TRALI). • Cardiomegaly (cardiothoracic ratio >0.55) and increased vascular pedicle width (>65 mm) suggest TACO rather than ALI (TRALI or possible TRALI).
Arterial blood gas analysis, arterial oxygen saturation (pulse oximetry)	• Test results quantify respiratory impairment. • PaO_2/FiO_2 <300 mm Hg (or O_2 saturation <90% on room air) with pulmonary edema that is not predominantly attributed to circulatory overload fulfills consensus conference criteria for ALI (TRALI or possible TRALI).

Table 2-4. Clinical Information That May Assist in Differential Diagnosis of Pulmonary Transfusion Reactions (Continued)

Clinical Information	Rationale
Hemodynamic monitoring: central venous and pulmonary artery pressures	Increases in central venous (>12-15 mm Hg) or pulmonary artery occlusion (>18-20 mm Hg) pressure at the time of the reaction suggest TACO.
Echocardiography	Systolic (ejection fraction <45%) or diastolic (E/E' >15) dysfunction suggest TACO or other cause of cardiogenic edema.
Pulmonary edema fluid	A ratio of pulmonary edema albumin over plasma albumin of >0.55 suggests ALI rather than hydrostatic (TACO) edema.
Natriuretic peptides: brain natriuretic peptide (BNP) and N-terminal prohormone BNP (NT-proBNP)	• Low values of BNP (<250 pg/mL) suggest ALI (TRALI or possible TRALI). • Increases in BNP or NT-proBNP >1.5 of pretransfusion values may suggest TACO.
Leukocyte and neutrophil count before and after the implicated transfusion	A sudden, short-lived drop in neutrophil or leukocyte count after the transfusion suggests TRALI.
Response to diuretic therapy	Rapid (minutes to hours) resolution of pulmonary edema after diuresis may suggest TACO.
Timing of the reaction in relation to transfusion and other potential risk factors	Sudden onset during or shortly after the transfusion is suggestive of a transfusion complication rather than a pulmonary complication related to another risk factor.

IgA = immunoglobulin A; TACO = transfusion-associated circulatory overload; TRALI = transfusion-related acute lung injury; ALI = acute lung injury; PaO_2/FiO_2 = partial pressure of oxygen in arterial blood/inspired oxygen concentration.

transfusion reactions not only will enhance the proper diagnosis and treatment of individual patients but also will allow blood centers to take appropriate actions regarding component safety and donor management.

Therapeutic Considerations of TRALI in the ICU

The mainstay of the treatment of TRALI is aggressive respiratory support, with supplemental oxygen and mechanical ventilation, if required.[5,8,36] Milder forms of TRALI require only the delivery of supplemental oxygen.[4,36] As noted earlier in this chapter, the separation of TACO from ALI (both TRALI and possible TRALI) is important because diuretics may be acutely helpful in TACO cases. Moreover, some TRALI reactions have an acute drop in blood pressure after the initial respiratory symptoms develop, and diuretics may be contraindicated in early TRALI reactions. After the lung injury has been established and hemodynamic instability has resolved, restrictive fluid management including diuretics may also be indicated in patients with TRALI in order to facilitate the resolution of pulmonary edema and to shorten the time on the ventilator.[54-56] Most patients with TACO and some patients with TRALI can be successfully managed by noninvasive mechanical ventilation. It is important to note that once the diagnosis of TRALI has been made, the treatment is the same as that used to manage ALI/ARDS or other etiologies. Relevant management includes low-tidal-volume invasive mechanical ventilation,[57] standardized sedation and weaning protocols,[58] and use of measures to prevent nosocomial complications that can improve the outcome of patients who require invasive mechanical ventilation.[56] The role of corticosteroid administration is controversial and is not currently a standard recommendation.[56,59,60] In the case of TRALI or possible TRALI, additional transfusions around the time of the acute event should be considered carefully. Blood components should not be withheld if they are likely to be efficacious, but a clear-cut indication should be defined, especially for higher plasma-volume components that may carry an increased risk for TRALI. To minimize exposure to biologic response modifiers immediately after the initial reaction, younger cell-containing blood components (RBCs ≤3 weeks and platelets 3 days old) or washed components may be considered.

Prevention

Designing an effective preventive strategy for TRALI should start off by improving awareness of the condition in the critical care and general medical community. Recognizing those at high risk for ALI and TRALI, such as those with severe sepsis, pneumonia, aspiration, and trauma, as well as avoiding liberal transfusion of these patients, is likely to reduce the occurrence regardless of the specific pathophysiologic mechanism. The introduction of bedside decision support for restrictive RBC transfusion has been associated with a decreased risk of ALI in mechanically ventilated patients without ALI at the outset.[21] Liberal transfusion of non-RBC components should also be avoided, particularly in patients without active bleeding.[19]

Considering the evidence provided in the clinical trial by Palfi et al[38] and the observational data in critically ill patients,[12,15,24] it would be a logical practice to exclude potentially alloimmunized donors (previously pregnant female donors) from the donor pool—in particular from the production of high-plasma-volume components such as FFP and platelets. (See Chapters 4 and 8.)

Because stored cellular blood components generate biologic response modifiers implicated in the pathogenesis of TRALI, some investigators have suggested that RBCs stored >2 weeks and platelets stored >3 days should not be transfused in those at risk for TRALI[49]; removing neutrophil priming agents (biologic response modifiers) by washing the blood components has also been suggested.[36] However, these suggestions have not achieved widespread consensus and are not supported by clinical data. The roles of patient predisposition, component storage time, preparation methods such as solvent/detergent-treatment of plasma, use of platelet-additive solutions, and washing of cellular blood components need to be defined better for effective preventive strategies.

Conclusion

The association between specific donor and transfusion characteristics and subsequent development of ALI in critically ill patients has important implications relative to both the etiology and the prevention of this syndrome. An international effort should be orchestrated to have a uniform approach to epidemiology, diagnosis, and prevention of ALI and TRALI in the critically ill. Over the past several years, more studies have been done on the subject of TRALI than before, indicating that the medical community is gradually increasing awareness of this important complication of blood transfusion. Several studies have shown that both massive and submassive (any) transfusions are independently associated with the development of ALI/ARDS. Although the evidence of a causal relationship between transfusion and ALI/ARDS remains limited, the burden of the problem forces an early implementation of potential preventive strategies, including a restrictive transfusion policy and the avoidance of plasma from donors with a high likelihood of alloimmunization.

References

1. Gajic O, Moore SB. Transfusion-related acute lung injury. Mayo Clin Proc 2005; 80:766-70.
2. Toy P, Popovsky MA, Abraham E, et al. Transfusion-related acute lung injury: Definition and review. Crit Care Med 2005;33:721-6.
3. Holness L, Knippen MA, Simmons L, Lachenbruch PA. Fatalities caused by TRALI. Transfus Med Rev 2004;18:184-8.
4. Kopko PM, Marshall CS, MacKenzie MR, et al. Transfusion-related acute lung injury: Report of a clinical look-back investigation. JAMA 2002;287:1968-71.

5.	Popovsky MA, Moore SB. Diagnostic and pathogenetic considerations in transfusion-related acute lung injury. Transfusion 1985;25:573-7.
6.	Sachs UJ, Hattar K, Weissmann N, et al. Antibody-induced neutrophil activation as a trigger for transfusion-related acute lung injury in an ex vivo rat lung model. Blood 2006;107:1217-19.
7.	Seeger W, Schneider U, Kreusler B, et al. Reproduction of transfusion-related acute lung injury in an ex vivo lung model. Blood 1990;76:1438-44.
8.	Silliman CC, Boshkov LK, Mehdizadehkashi Z, et al. Transfusion-related acute lung injury: Epidemiology and a prospective analysis of etiologic factors. Blood 2003;101:454-62.
9.	Silliman CC, Voelkel NF, Allard JD, et al. Plasma and lipids from stored packed red blood cells cause acute lung injury in an animal model. J Clin Invest 1998;101:1458-67.
10.	Boffard KD, Riou B, Warren B, et al. Recombinant Factor VIIa as adjunctive therapy for bleeding control in severely injured trauma patients: Two parallel randomized, placebo-controlled, double-blind clinical trials. J Trauma 2005;59:8-15.
11.	Hébert PC, Wells G, Blajchman MA, et al. A multicenter, randomized, controlled clinical trial of transfusion requirements in critical care. Transfusion Requirements in Critical Care Investigators, Canadian Critical Care Trials Group. N Engl J Med 1999;340:409-17.
12.	Gajic O, Yilmaz M, Iscimen R, et al. Transfusion from male-only versus female donors in critically ill recipients of high plasma volume components. Crit Care Med 2007;35:1645-8.
13.	Rana R, Afessa B, Keegan MT, et al. Evidence-based red cell transfusion in the critically ill: Quality improvement using computerized physician order entry. Crit Care Med 2006;34:1892-7.
14.	Gajic O, Rana R, Mendez JL, et al. Acute lung injury after blood transfusion in mechanically ventilated patients. Transfusion 2004;44:1468-74.
15.	Gajic O, Rana R, Winters JL, et al. Transfusion-related acute lung injury in the critically ill: Prospective nested case-control study. Am J Respir Crit Care Med 2007;176:886-91.
16.	Gong MN, Thompson BT, Williams P, et al. Clinical predictors of and mortality in acute respiratory distress syndrome: Potential role of red cell transfusion. Crit Care Med 2005;33:1191-8.
17.	Silverboard H, Aisiku I, Martin G, et al. The role of acute blood transfusion in the development of acute respiratory distress syndrome in patients with severe trauma. J Trauma 2005;59:717-23.
18.	Zilberberg M, Carter C, Lefebvre P, et al. Red blood cell transfusions and the risk of acute respiratory disease syndrome among the critically ill: A cohort study. Crit Care 2007;11:R63.
19.	Dara S, Rana R, Afessa B, et al. Fresh Frozen Plasma transfusion in critically ill medical patients with coagulopathy. Crit Care Med 2005;33:2667-71.
20.	Gajic O, Dara SI, Mendez JL, et al. Ventilator-associated lung injury in patients without acute lung injury at the onset of mechanical ventilation. Crit Care Med 2004;32:1817-24.

21. Yilmaz M, Keegan MT, Iscimen R, et al. Toward the prevention of acute lung injury: Protocol-guided limitation of large tidal volume ventilation and inappropriate transfusion. Crit Care Med 2007;35:1660-6.

22. Khan H, Belsher J, Yilmaz M, et al. Fresh-Frozen Plasma and platelet transfusions are associated with development of acute lung injury in critically ill medical patients. Chest 2007;131:1308-14.

23. Rana R, Fernandez-Perez ER, Khan SA, et al. Transfusion-related acute lung injury and pulmonary edema in critically ill patients: A retrospective study. Transfusion 2006;46:1478-83.

24. Wright SE, Snowden CP, Athey S, et al. Acute lung injury after ruptured abdominal aortic aneurysm repair: The effect of excluding donations from females from the production of fresh frozen plasma. Crit Care Med 2008;36: 1796-802.

25. Gajic O, Gropper MA, Hubmayr RD. Pulmonary edema after transfusion: How to differentiate transfusion-associated circulatory overload from transfusion-related acute lung injury. Crit Care Med 2006;34(Suppl 5):S109-13.

26. Kleinman S, Caulfield T, Chan P, et al. Toward an understanding of transfusion-related acute lung injury: Statement of a consensus panel. Transfusion 2004; 44:1774-89.

27. Barnard RD. Indiscriminate transfusion: A critique of case reports illustrating hypersensitivity reactions. N Y State J Med 1951;51:2399-402.

28. Popovsky MA, Abel MD, Moore SB. Transfusion-related acute lung injury associated with passive transfer of antileukocyte antibodies. Am Rev Respir Dis 1983;128:185-9.

29. Popovsky MA, Davenport RD. Transfusion-related acute lung injury: Femme fatale? Transfusion 2001;41:312-5.

30. Pepe PE, Potkin RT, Reus DH, et al. Clinical predictors of the adult respiratory distress syndrome. Am J Surg 1982;144:124-30.

31. Hudson LD, Milberg JA, Anardi D, Maunder RJ. Clinical risks for development of the acute respiratory distress syndrome. Am J Respir Crit Care Med 1995; 151:293-301.

32. Belsher J, Khan H, Gajic O. Transfusion as a risk factor for ALI and ARDS. In: Vincent JL, ed. Yearbook of intensive care and emergency medicine. Berlin: Springer Science and Business Media, 2006:289-96.

33. Gong MN, Wei Z, Xu LL, et al. Polymorphism in the surfactant protein-B gene, gender, and the risk of direct pulmonary injury and ARDS. Chest 2004;125: 203-11.

34. Croce MA, Tolley EA, Claridge JA, Fabian TC. Transfusions result in pulmonary morbidity and death after a moderate degree of injury. J Trauma 2005; 59:19-23.

35. Salman SS, Fernández Pérez ER, Stubbs JR, Gajic O. The practice of platelet transfusion in the intensive care unit. J Intensive Care Med 2007;22:105-10.

36. Silliman CC, Ambruso DR, Boshkov LK. Transfusion-related acute lung injury. Blood 2005;105:2266-73.

37. Bux J, Sachs UJ. The pathogenesis of transfusion-related acute lung injury (TRALI). Br J Haematol 2007;136:788-99.

38. Palfi M, Berg S, Ernerudh J, Berlin G. A randomized controlled trial of transfusion-related acute lung injury: Is plasma from multiparous blood donors dangerous? Transfusion 2001;41:317-22.

39. Insunza A, Romon I, Gonzalez-Ponte ML, et al. Implementation of a strategy to prevent TRALI in a regional blood centre. Transfus Med 2004;14:157-64.

40. Bray RA, Harris SB, Josephson CD, et al. Unappreciated risk factors for transplant patients: HLA antibodies in blood components. Hum Immunol 2004; 65:240-4.

41. Reiter CD, Wang X, Tanus-Santos JE, et al. Cell-free hemoglobin limits nitric oxide bioavailability in sickle-cell disease. Nat Med 2002;8:1383-9.

42. Rivers E, Nguyen B, Havstad S, et al. Early goal-directed therapy in the treatment of severe sepsis and septic shock. N Engl J Med 2001;345:1368-77.

43. Zilberberg MD, Epstein SK. Acute lung injury in the medical ICU: Comorbid conditions, age, etiology, and hospital outcome. Am J Respir Crit Care Med 1998;157:1159-64.

44. Rana R, Vlahakis NE, Daniels CE, et al. B-type natriuretic peptide in the assessment of acute lung injury and cardiogenic pulmonary edema. Crit Care Med 2006;34:1941-6.

45. Churg A, Muller NL, Silva CI, Wright JL. Acute exacerbation (acute lung injury of unknown cause) in UIP and other forms of fibrotic interstitial pneumonias. Am J Surg Pathol 2007;31:277-84.

46. Silliman CC, Paterson AJ, Dickey WO, et al. The association of biologically active lipids with the development of transfusion-related acute lung injury: A retrospective study. Transfusion 1997;37:719-26.

47. Covin RB, Ambruso DR, England KM, et al. Hypotension and acute pulmonary insufficiency following transfusion of autologous red blood cells during surgery: A case report and review of the literature. Transfus Med 2004;14: 375-83.

48. Bernard GR, Artigas A, Brigham KL, et al. The American-European Consensus Conference on ARDS. Definitions, mechanisms, relevant outcomes, and clinical trial coordination. Am J Respir Crit Care Med 1994;149:818-24.

49. Goldman M, Webert KE, Arnold DM, et al. Proceedings of a consensus conference: Towards an understanding of TRALI. Transfus Med Rev 2005;19:2-31.

50. Popovsky MA. Transfusion and the lung: Circulatory overload and acute lung injury. Vox Sang 2004;87(Suppl 2):62-5.

51. Bierbaum BE, Callaghan JJ, Galante JO, et al. An analysis of blood management in patients having a total hip or knee arthroplasty. J Bone Joint Surg Am 1999;81:2-10.

52. Ryffel B, Couillin I, Maillet I, et al. Histamine scavenging attenuates endotoxin-induced acute lung injury. Ann N Y Acad Sci 2005;1056:197-205.

53. Swigris JJ, Brown KK. Acute interstitial pneumonia and acute exacerbations of idiopathic pulmonary fibrosis. Semin Respir Crit Care Med 2006;27:659-67.

54. The National Heart, Lung, and Blood Institute Acute Respiratory Distress Syndrome (ARDS) Clinical Trials Network. Comparison of two fluid-management strategies in acute lung injury. N Engl J Med 2006;354:2564-75.

55. The National Heart, Lung, and Blood Institute Acute Respiratory Distress Syndrome (ARDS) Clinical Trials Network. Pulmonary-artery versus central

venous catheter to guide treatment of acute lung injury. N Engl J Med 2006;354:2213-24.

56. Wheeler AP, Bernard GR. Acute lung injury and the acute respiratory distress syndrome: A clinical review. Lancet 2007;369:1553-64.

57. The Acute Respiratory Distress Syndrome Network. Ventilation with lower tidal volumes as compared with traditional tidal volumes for acute lung injury and the acute respiratory distress syndrome. N Engl J Med 2000;342:1301-8.

58. Kress JP, Pohlman AS, O'Connor MF, Hall JB. Daily interruption of sedative infusions in critically ill patients undergoing mechanical ventilation. N Engl J Med 2000;342:1471-7.

59. The National Heart, Lung, and Blood Institute Acute Respiratory Distress Syndrome (ARDS) Clinical Trials Network. Efficacy and safety of corticosteroids for persistent acute respiratory distress syndrome. N Engl J Med 2006;354:1671-84.

60. Meduri GU, Golden E, Freire AX, et al. Methylprednisolone infusion in early severe ARDS: Results of a randomized controlled trial. Chest 2007;131:954-63.

In: Kleinman S, Popovsky MA, eds.
TRALI: Mechanisms, Management, and Prevention
Bethesda, MD: AABB Press, 2008

3

Pathophysiology of TRALI

JÜRGEN BUX, MD, PhD, AND
ULRICH J.H. SACHS, MD, PhD

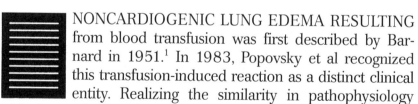 NONCARDIOGENIC LUNG EDEMA RESULTING from blood transfusion was first described by Barnard in 1951.[1] In 1983, Popovsky et al recognized this transfusion-induced reaction as a distinct clinical entity. Realizing the similarity in pathophysiology with the syndrome of acute lung injury (ALI) seen in critically ill patients, they coined the term "transfusion-related acute lung injury" (TRALI).[2] Two years later, Popovsky and Moore analyzed

Jürgen Bux, MD, PhD, Chief Medical Director, German Red Cross Blood Donor Service West, Hagen, Germany, and Ulrich J.H. Sachs, MD, PhD, Head, The Platelet and Granulocyte Laboratory, Institute for Clinical Immunology and Transfusion Medicine, Justus Liebig University, Giessen, Germany a series of 36 well-defined TRALI patients.[3] In this study, the presence of leukocyte (ie, neutrophil and HLA) antibodies was reported in the blood from 89% of the implicated donors. These reports are early milestones in identifying the mechanisms responsible for TRALI; it has been thanks to hemovigilance schemes, clinical findings, histopathology, and experimental work that an understanding of the condition has increased significantly in the past 10 years. Two early observations are still valid: TRALI shares a common pathophysiology with ALI seen in critically ill patients, and leukocyte antibodies are the most relevant inducers of TRALI.

Acute Lung Injury and TRALI

ALI is the result of a capillary endothelial leak that allows fluid to pass from the pulmonary vessels into the interstitial space and, subsequently, into the alveoli. As distinct from hydrostatic edema with a protein-poor transudate, pulmonary edema in ALI is an exudate with a high-protein content. Numerous stimuli have been reported to contribute to the development of ALI, including transfusion. Whereas, in some cases, the transfusion event appears to be only one of several factors present, in other cases, it may constitute the only probable cause of lung injury.

ALI and TRALI share a common clinical picture, the difference being that, in TRALI, ALI is connected to a transfusion event in a temporal and causative manner. Significant similarities are also seen in histopathology, including the following:

- Interstitial and often intra-alveolar edema.[3-9]
- Sequestration of neutrophils in the pulmonary microvasculature.
- Extravasation of neutrophils into the interstitial and air spaces.[4-6,9]
- Hyaline membranes and destruction of the pulmonary architecture in severe cases.[4,6]

A consistent finding in TRALI is the presence of increased numbers of neutrophils in the pulmonary capillary vasculature and the small pulmonary vessels.[8,9] A positive correlation between the degree of capillary leukostasis and the amount of proteinaceous fluid in the alveolar air spaces has been demonstrated.[8,9] In electron-microscopic pictures, neutrophils were degranulated and focally in direct contact with denuded stretches of the capillary wall.[9] From these observations, it appears that the neutrophil is central to the occurrence of lung damage in TRALI.

Although, in ALI of the severely ill patient, it is difficult to elucidate how the neutrophil is activated to cause damage to the lungs, it is clear that, in TRALI, neutrophil-priming or neutrophil-activating mediators must be present in transfused blood components.

Evidence for an Antibody-Related Etiology

The relationship between TRALI and leukocyte antibodies in donor plasma was first noted by Brittingham who reported that leukoagglutinins present in the plasma of a multiply transfused patient induced acute pulmonary reactions when transfused into a volunteer.[10] Severe pulmonary edema was similarly induced in a healthy volunteer who received an experimental gamma globulin concentrate deliberately prepared from plasma that contained leukocyte-reactive antibodies.[11] A third demonstration of the effect of leukocyte antibodies was reported after a volunteer was infused with 100 mL of plasma from a donor known to have HLA Class II antibodies but no neutrophil-specific or HLA Class I antibodies. The transfusion resulted in a moderate degree of ALI.[12]

In addition to these three cases of TRALI resulting from the experimental transfusion of plasma containing leukocyte antibodies to healthy volunteers, there are numerous case reports of TRALI in which a transfused unit has been found to contain antibodies reactive with recipient leukocytes. In two large series of TRALI cases where pulmonary infiltrates were apparent in chest radiographs, leukocyte antibodies in the donor of a transfused blood component were detected in 61% to 90% of cases.[3,13] Animal models have provided confirmation of this antibody-mediated mechanism of TRALI[14-16] (a detailed discussion follows later in this chapter). Besides leukocyte antibodies, nonimmune neutrophil-priming substances formed during platelet and red cell storage have been identified as alternative mediators of TRALI.[17] However, it must be pointed out that neither leukocyte antibodies nor nonimmune TRALI mediators present in blood components will necessarily cause TRALI in the recipient. It is well known that the development of ALI depends on the individual predisposition of the patient; clinical and experimental evidence that the same applies to TRALI has recently been compiled in the threshold model of TRALI.[18]

Threshold Model of TRALI

The threshold model[18] suggests that the neutrophil is central to the pathogenesis of TRALI and that activation of the neutrophil requires sufficient stimuli from one or more sources to reach a certain threshold, at which point full cellular activation and lung damage will ensue. Accordingly, where the stimulus to neutrophil activation is sufficient, lung damage can occur in an otherwise healthy individual with no other likely cause of lung injury. Evidence for this finding comes from reports of TRALI in transfused volunteers, as well as from reports where plasma has been used for clinical reasons in otherwise healthy individuals. These cases are the minority because most patients receiving transfusions—especially the transfusion of plasma—have significant comorbidities, which may also affect the lung tissues. It has been suggested that TRALI will be more common in such patients.[17] Early reports noted that most patients with TRALI had recently undergone surgery, suggesting that this in itself was a sufficient additional stimulus in many cases.[3] Experimental evidence has been provided by ex-vivo rat lung model studies in which the infusion of neutrophil antibodies was able to induce TRALI in the presence of a high antigen load.[15] Here, the addition of N-formylmethionyleucyl-phenylalanine (fMLP) as an additional mediator mimicking the presence of bacterial infection could elicit TRALI even if the antigen load was low. Somewhat comparably, bioactive lipids were able to induce lung injury in rats only after the rat had received an injection of lipopolysaccharides (LPS).[19]

The proposed threshold model of TRALI (see Fig 3-1) summarizes these factors as the individual predisposition of the transfusion recipient on the one hand and as the strength of transfusion-related mediators (eg, antibodies, lipids) on the other hand. Individual predisposition covers both constitutive (genetic) and comorbidity-related factors (eg, infection, disseminated intravascular coagulation, aspiration, shock). Depending on the magnitude of the neutrophil response, lung damage can be mild or severe, with corresponding clinical effects.

Neutrophil Transit through the Lungs

All circulating blood has to pass through the lungs. Thus, all blood leukocytes have to travel through the pulmonary microvessels. The alveolar capillary bed is a complex interconnecting network of billions of short capillary segments. On their way from arteriole to venule, leukocytes encounter more than 50 capillary segments, and approximately half of the pulmonary capillaries are narrower than the diameter of a spherically shaped neutrophil (6-8 µm). Thus, neutrophils will often encounter capillary segments that force them to pause, deform, and assume a "sausage" shape before squeezing through the narrow capillary segment. Consequently, the transit time of neutrophils through the pulmonary capillary bed is affected mainly by their deformation time. In contrast to the rapidly deformable

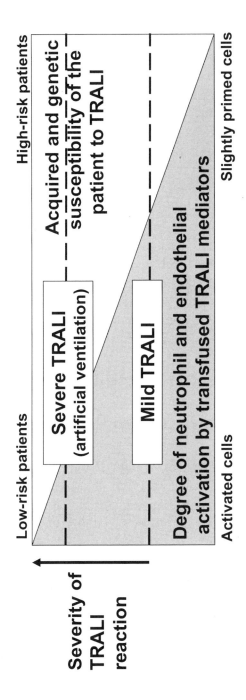

Figure 3-1. Threshold model of TRALI. The occurrence and severity of TRALI depend mainly on the patient's susceptibility to develop TRALI and on the degree of neutrophil and pulmonary endothelium priming/activation by mediators present in blood components. In patients with a genetic defect for the inactivation of inflammatory mediators or with an underlying disease affecting the lung, a weak stimulus might be sufficient for the development of TRALI. However, neutrophil-activating mediators in blood components, such as leukoagglutinins, are able to elicit TRALI even in healthy individuals. In TRALI with mild symptoms but new bilateral lung infiltrates in the chest x-ray, oxygen support is sufficient, whereas severe TRALI cases are characterized by the requirement of mechanical ventilation. (Modified with permission from Bux and Sachs.[18])

red cells, neutrophils require much longer transit times.[20] The increased transit time also accounts for the physiologic neutrophil accumulation (ie, the "marginated pool" in the lungs)[21]; the pulmonary circulation contains about 28% of the blood neutrophil pool at any given time.[22]

The principal site of leukocyte transmigration in the lung—at sites of inflammation—is the capillary bed and not, as in other organs, the postcapillary venule.[23-25] Because neutrophils do not roll in lung capillaries, the conventional model of neutrophil tethering, rolling, and arresting on an inflamed endothelium is not applicable to lung capillaries.[26] Instead, a stimulus-induced decrease in deformability is thought to be important for neutrophil sequestration in the lung as a result of an inflammatory challenge, and it likely replaces the role of selectin-mediated rolling in stopping neutrophils within capillaries.[21,26,27] Activated neutrophils lose their ability to deform mainly because of intracellular polymerization of actin filaments. In contrast, maintenance of sequestered neutrophils in the microvasculature and their subsequent transendothelial migration are apparently influenced by adhesion molecules. The pulmonary microvasculature seems to preferentially retain cells that express high levels of L-selectin. Furthermore, mechanical trapping occurs together with neutrophil adhesion to the endothelial surface because mediator-induced decreases in neutrophil deformability are temporally correlated with a conformational change of β_2-integrins from nonadhesive to adhesive. Intercellular adhesion molecule 2 (ICAM-2, or CD102), a ligand of the β_2-integrin CD11b/CD18, is constitutively expressed on endothelial cells and appears to play a role in neutrophil transendothelial migration.[28] After activation, endothelial cells up-regulate ICAM-1, a major ligand for CD11b/CD18. Transendothelial migration occurs primarily by penetrating interendothelial junctions at bicellular or tricellular corners of endothelial cells, although there is an alternative transcellular route.[26] Platelet endothelial cell adhesion molecule 1 (PECAM-1, or CD31), junctional adhesion molecules (JAMs), vascular endothelial (VE)-cadherin, and CD99 are thought to regulate neutrophil transendothelial migration.[29]

Mechanisms Leading to Lung Damage in TRALI

The vascular endothelium and the alveolar epithelium form the two alveolar-capillary barriers. Under physiologic conditions, the endothelial barrier is more permeable than the epithelial one. Fluid filtered by the capillaries enters the alveolar interstitial space through small gaps between capillary endothelial cells, but it does not enter the alveolar space because alveolar epithelial cells are connected by very tight junctions. From the alveolar interstitium, the fluid moves into the peribronchovascular space, where it is removed by the lymphatics and returned to the systemic circulation.[30] Increased transendothelial fluid filtration is the hallmark of cardiogenic or volume overload lung edema. By contrast, noncardiogenic lung edema is caused by an increase in vascular permeability, resulting in an increased flux of fluid and protein into the lung interstitium and air spaces. The extent of epithelial injury is of critical importance to recovery from this dysfunction.

TRALI affects primarily the endothelial barrier, which might explain why the mortality in TRALI (6% to 12%) is relatively low when compared to typical cases of acute respiratory distress syndrome (ARDS) as a result of aspiration, pneumonia, trauma, or sepsis (30% to 40%).

Activation of the Neutrophil

Neutrophil priming and activation are of central importance in the pathogenesis of TRALI as indicated by histologic studies showing marked neutrophil sequestration in the lungs. After contact with activating stimuli, neutrophils will respond by aggregation, by phagocytosis, by the release of preformed enzymes and proteins from the intracellular granules, and by de-novo synthesis of a range of ephemeral, but highly toxic, reactive oxygen species (ROS). However, circulating (resting) neutrophils do not express their full microbicidal capacity when challenged with biologic activating agents unless the neutrophils have first been primed.

Priming refers to a process whereby the response of neutrophils to an activating stimulus is potentiated. Priming of neutrophils promotes 1) cell stiffening as a result of the polymerization of actin fibers in the cytoskeleton, 2) adhesivity caused by conformational proadhesive changes in the β_2-integrins, 3) shedding of L-selectins, 4) clustering of relevant surface receptors (eg, FcγRIIa and β_2-integrins), 5) release of toxic granule enzymes, and, most important, 6) formation of the nicotinamide adenine dinucleotide phosphate (NADPH) oxidase complex necessary for the synthesis of cytotoxic ROS. The release of ROS is enhanced up to 20-fold by prior exposure of the cell to a priming agent.[31] Priming agents do not elicit effector functions on their own except when they are applied at very high concentrations or encounter already primed cells. Primed neutrophils can already be present in patients as a consequence of the underlying disease.

A large percentage of patients who have developed TRALI had recent surgery. Patients with active infection, cardiovascular disease, and leukemia have been identified to be at risk for TRALI.[6,32,33] These observations are in accordance with in-vivo evidence from studies demonstrating that surgical procedures and active infections induce neutrophil priming in patients.[34-36]

Neutrophil priming can be induced by a variety of agents that are released either by dying or necrotic cells or by stimulated endothelial cells, monocytes, and lymphocytes, including platelet-activating factor (PAF),[37] tumor necrosis factor alpha (TNF-α),[38] interleukin (IL)-8,[39] granulocyte-macrophage colony-stimulating factor (GM-CSF),[40] and interferon (IFN)-γ.[41] Neutrophils can also be primed by infectious agents[42] and bacteria-derived lipopolysaccharide (LPS).[31] Despite these physiologic observations, it should be kept in mind that definitively linking TRALI to any specific clinical event or condition needs valid denominator data gathered in appropriate clinical trials, a prerequisite that has not yet been fulfilled.

In response to priming agents, neutrophils experience stiffening, which augments the mechanical retention of neutrophils in the pulmonary microvasculature (sequestration) and prolongs the process of neutrophils squeezing through narrow capillaries.[43] Prolonged close contact of the primed neutrophil with the endothelium facilitates cellular cross-talk in which transmembrane receptors and released mediators of each cell type can easily influence the other. The sequestered primed neutrophils can now be activated to express their full microbicidal activity by neutrophil-stimulating substances (cytokines, bioactive lipids) and neutrophil-binding antibodies present in the blood bag.

Exogenous TRALI mediators can also activate circulating preprimed neutrophils of the patient and can induce their active aggregation. Neutrophil aggregates will then be trapped in the pulmonary microvasculature (the first capillary network they pass through), where activated cells release deleterious enzymes and toxic ROS.

As mentioned earlier, priming substances can also induce full activation of resting neutrophils when applied at high concentrations. In addition to chemokines and cytokines, cross-linking antibodies to neutrophil surface receptors have been demonstrated to prime neutrophils[44,45] and to cause neutrophil activation either by themselves or in concert with nonimmune neutrophil priming substances.[46,47] Research has demonstrated that antibodies to antigens on neutrophils involved in TRALI cases are able to prime and even to activate neutrophils as well.[15,48-50] This finding explains why even completely healthy individuals can develop TRALI after neutrophil-antibody infusion.[11] Direct activation of resting neutrophils is typical for so-called leukoagglutinins of the IgG class. These antibodies induce active neutrophil aggregation, whereas passive cell agglutination is restricted to antibodies of the IgM class.[51]

Activation of Pulmonary Endothelial Cells

Priming and activation of pulmonary endothelial cells can also constitute the primary triggers for TRALI, especially during inflammatory processes, whereby various substances are released that have been identified as endothelial cell activators, such as TNF-α and IL-1β. The activated endothelium becomes procoagulant, proadhesive, vasoconstrictive, and proapoptotic. Proadhesivity is the result of an up-regulation of adhesion molecules, including P-selectin, ligands for L-selectin, and ICAM-1.[52-55] Circulating (resting) neutrophils may get directly "captured" through adhesion molecules of the activated endothelium or in conjunction with platelet-endothelial interactions.[56-58] Captured neutrophils will incorporate selectin-dependent and selectin-independent signals [eg, by endothelial PAF, leukotriene B4 (LTB4), and IL-8] as well as extracellular proinflammatory stimuli to achieve a primed status.[59] Once primed, neutrophils can respond with their full microbicidal arsenal when exposed to mediators present in transfused blood components that would otherwise only induce priming.

Stimulation of endothelial cells is a prerequisite for TRALI induction after infusion of bioactive lipids.[19,60] In a rat lung model, only rats pretreated with LPS to simulate active infection developed TRALI after the transfusion of plasma containing bioactive lipids that can develop during the storage of blood components.[61] Lungs pretreated with buffer/saline instead of LPS did not show evidence of TRALI.

Exogenous stimuli present in the transfused blood can also stimulate the pulmonary endothelium. One interesting example of TRALI caused by antibody-mediated endothelial cell activation was reported in a patient who underwent a single lung transplantation.[62] After transfusion of an RBC unit containing an antibody to HLA-B44, the patient became dyspneic and a chest x-ray revealed a white-out of the transplanted lung. The HLA-B44 antigen was expressed on the transplanted lung but not on the patient's own tissues because he was typed as HLA-B44 negative. Obviously, the TRALI reaction was triggered by antibody binding to the endothelium of the transplanted lung. Looney and coworkers[16] presented in-vivo data on the mechanism of endothelial cell-dependent TRALI in a mouse model, which indicated that HLA antibody-mediated endothelial cell activation may contribute to the development of TRALI.

Neutrophil/Endothelial Cell Interplay

The interplay between neutrophils and endothelial cells contributes largely to lung damage. Neutrophils respond to endothelial cell-derived mediators by activating and expressing integrins and by releasing proinflammatory mediators, granule enzmyes, and proteins, as well as ROS. The released mediators activate the endothelial cells that mobilize selectins, up-regulate adhesion proteins, and produce proinflammatory mediators, thereby enhancing neutrophil adhesion, priming, and activation. It is in this interplay that the endothelium barrier breaks down and allows extravasation of proteinaceous fluid and, later, of neutrophils. ROS play a crucial role in this process. In an animal model of lung injury, a blockade of ROS protected the lungs from edema and vascular leak.[63] Neutrophil-specific antibodies, as well as bioactive lipids, have been demonstrated to prime the respiratory burst of the neutrophil.[6,15] In addition to disintegration of the plasma membrane, ROS are known to induce PECAM-1 on endothelial cells, an important molecule for transendothelial migration of neutrophils.[64] In fact, up-regulation of PECAM-1 has been observed on endothelial cells of pulmonary vasculature from a patient who died from TRALI.[65]

Monocytes

Monocyte-mediated neutrophil priming/activation has been suggested as a possible mechanism for the pathogenesis of HLA Class II antibody-induced TRALI.[66] Monocytes expressing the cognate HLA Class II antigen are probably primed by the antibodies, and interaction of the primed monocytes with activated endothelial cells induces the monocytes to release neutrophil-attracting and -stimulating mediators, such as LTB4.[67]

Participation of Platelets and the Coagulation Cascade

Platelets and the coagulation cascade are known to be implicated in ALI. There is evidence that microvascular thrombosis is an early event in the development of ALI/ARDS.[26] Tissue factor expressed by circulating monocytes and endothelial cells under proinflammatory conditions might play a central role because activated tissue factor also induces the expression of several proinflammatory genes.[68] Furthermore, the blocking of platelet-neutrophil aggregation has been found in a mouse model to reverse ALI.[58] However, the contribution of hemostasis to the development of TRALI has not yet been carefully investigated.

Participation of the Complement System

Complement activation has been found to contribute to ALI/ARDS after cardiopulmonary bypass.[69] Although in one animal model of antibody-mediated TRALI, the presence of complement was necessary for TRALI induction,[14] the exact role of complement in the development of TRALI remains to be elucidated.[18]

Cell priming and activation events in TRALI are summarized in Fig 3-2.

Priming and Activating Substances Present in Blood Components

It is likely that substances contained in blood components can induce TRALI by one of several mechanisms: by priming and/or activating neutrophils, by activating endothelial cells of the pulmonary vasculature, or by stimulating monocytes.

Leukocyte Antibodies

Antibodies to HLA Class I and II antigens and to human neutrophil antigens (HNA) have all been implicated as causing TRALI. Current hemovigilance data suggest that the majority of

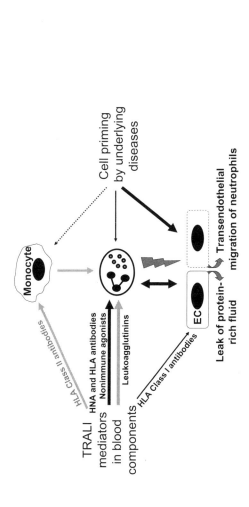

Figure 3-2. Cell priming and activation in TRALI. Neutrophils and endothelial cells (EC) of the pulmonary capillaries are crucial to the pathogenesis of TRALI. Priming or activation of these cells can be caused by the patient's underlying disease and by antibodies and nonimmune mediators in blood components. Most frequently, transfused mediators will encounter pulmonary endothelial cells and neutrophils primed by comorbidity. This encounter results in neutrophil activation, release of harmful enzymes, and reactive oxygen species that damage the endothelium. The disruption of the endothelial barrier leads to leakage of protein-rich fluid into the alveoli and to neutrophil transmigration. In some cases, leukocyte antibodies can already activate neutrophils so they injure the lung capillaries even if the pulmonary endothelium has not been primed by the patient's underlying disease. This is thought to occur after the transfusion of components containing high amounts of neutrophil-aggregating antibodies, the so-called leukoagglutinins.

cases are associated with HLA antibodies, mainly directed against Class II antigens. Antibodies to HNA are less common, but they have been often implicated in severe and fatal TRALI cases.

In a large series of TRALI cases, where pulmonary infiltrates were apparent in chest radiographs, leukocyte antibodies were detected in 61% to 90% of the cases, with the causative antibody being identified in the donor of the transfused component.[3,13] As early as 1957, Brittingham reported that leukocyte antibodies can induce posttransfusion pulmonary reactions in volunteers[10]: a healthy volunteer received plasma from two patients that contained a weak leukoagglutinin, and a mild respiratory reaction occurred after both transfusions. Subsequently, the same volunteer received 50 mL of whole blood from an alloimmunized patient with strong leukoagglutinins and developed neutropenia, fever, and a marked respiratory reaction with bilateral pulmonary infiltrates on a chest x-ray. A similar reaction occurred when a leukemic patient was injected with 10 mL of sterile serum obtained from a patient with a strong leukoagglutinin. Severe pulmonary edema was induced in a healthy volunteer who received an experimental gamma globulin concentrate prepared from plasma containing leukocyte-reactive antibodies.[11]

Although the antigens recognized by the antibodies in these reports were not well characterized, it appears that some leukocyte antibodies, especially leukoagglutinins, in transfused components are capable of inducing TRALI in a "one-step" reaction, probably because they are strong enough to induce both neutrophil priming and activation. Although these antibodies are often referred to as leukoagglutinins, most of them induce active neutrophil aggregation and do not passively agglutinate neutrophils. Aggregation refers to an active process where, subsequent to antibody binding, the neutrophils become activated and clump. In contrast, agglutination represents a passive mechanism of neutrophil clustering, a reaction restricted to antibodies of the IgM class.

From a pathogenetic point of view, it is necessary to distinguish between antibodies that recognize HNA, expressed on neutrophils (but not on the endothelium), and antibodies that recognize HLA Class I, expressed on both the neutrophil and the endothelium.

Antibodies to Human Neutrophil Antigens

Serologic workups of TRALI patients identified antibodies to HNA in a number of cases[70-73]; descriptions of HNA and their implication in TRALI have been published elsewhere.[74] It is known to the authors that one of these antibodies, a neutrophil agglutinin directed against HNA-3a, induced acute dyspnea even in a healthy human volunteer after injection of a small volume of donor plasma. Details of the mechanism were studied in an ex-vivo rabbit lung model.[14] Severe vascular leakage was reproduced in isolated rabbit lungs by the application of HNA-3a antibodies. In the presence of HNA-3a-positive neutrophils and complement, severe lung edema occurred after a latent period of 3 to 6 hours. In contrast, no such reaction was noted in the absence of HNA-3a antibodies, HNA-3a-positive neutrophils, or a complement source. From these experiments, it was concluded that leukoagglutinating antibodies and concomitant complement activation are key players in the initiation of TRALI. However, complement activation has not been found to be a prerequisite for antibody-mediated TRALI induction in other ex-vivo experiments.[15] It seems reasonable to speculate that antibodies to HNA-3a were also capable of priming and activating neutrophils. It has been demonstrated recently that HNA-3a antibodies are able to prime neutrophils in vitro,[49,50] as are antibodies to HNA-4a and HNA-2a.[15,48]

Antibodies directed against the neutrophil-specific surface marker CD177 (HNA-2a) were recently used by the authors to demonstrate that TRALI induction in an ex-vivo rat lung model is dependent on the density of the cognate antigen and can be efficiently enhanced by the addition of fMLP, a substance that mimics the activity of bacterially derived peptides and is used to simulate active infection.[15] HNA-2a expression is heterogeneous in humans, with HNA-2a frequently being expressed on either a large subpopulation (70%) or a small subpopulation (30%) of neutrophils, varying from individual to individual. The authors used neutrophils from each group of healthy donors in an ex-vivo rat lung model, and application of the corresponding antibody induced TRALI only if CD177 was present on the majority of neutrophils. Obviously, under these conditions, neutrophil-antibody interaction was capable of fully activating the cells. In contrast, if CD177 was present on the minority of cells, no TRALI reaction could be induced by antibody addition. However, if fMLP was added, TRALI induction was promoted in the presence of neutrophils from individuals expressing CD177 on more than 70% of their cells, as well as those expressing CD177 on less than 30% of their cells.

These findings indicate that additional stimuli can overcome the inability of a stimulus to activate neutrophils. Thus, it can be deduced from these findings that, if antibodies are present in a blood component, they may be able to induce TRALI in an otherwise healthy individual (including healthy volunteers) whenever the antigen/antibody ratio allows appropriate neutrophil activation. These findings are also in agreement with reports from healthy volunteers developing TRALI after antibody infusion.[10,11] However, if an individual's neutrophils encounter additional stimuli, it appears that TRALI could develop more readily.

HLA Antibodies

Although HLA antibodies are frequently reported in TRALI cases, only a few studies have investigated the mechanisms by which these antibodies can induce a TRALI reaction. In contrast to HNA antibodies, HLA Class I antigens are present on the surface of endothelial cells. Transfusion of a major histocompatibility complex (MHC) Class I monoclonal antibody to mice expressing the cognate antigen induced TRALI and acute peripheral blood neutropenia. Mice lacking neutrophils and mice lacking the Fcγ receptor were resistant to MHC Class I antibody-induced TRALI. Transfer of wild-type neutrophils into FcRγ$^{-/-}$ mice resulted in TRALI after antibody infusion. This model is consistent with binding of the antibody directly to endothelial cells, in the first vascular bed encountered after injection, and recruitment of neutrophils through binding of the immunoglobulin Fc portion to the neutrophil Fcγ receptor. The protection observed in FcRγ$^{-/-}$ mice argues against direct neutrophil activation by the antibody. In this study, it would appear that a direct (Fab-dependent) interaction between MHC Class I antibodies and the neutrophils did not contribute to the TRALI reaction. One limitation of this model is that a monoclonal antibody was used, which probably was unable to induce neutrophil priming or activation, or both.

Unfortunately, there is no systematic evaluation of HLA Class I antibodies with regard to their priming activity. However, it is known that some HLA antibodies, such as anti-HLA-A2, can induce neutrophil aggregation in vitro, whereas many others cannot. Because neutrophil aggregation implies neutrophil activation, these HLA antibodies must be able to prime and to activate neutrophils. In addition, it has to be kept in mind that antibodies of the same specificity are not always functionally alike, as the authors have demonstrated for human antibodies recognizing HNA-4a on CD11b. Some of these antibodies were capable of inducing the respiratory burst reaction, whereas others were not, although their serologic specificity was identical.[48] Thus, it cannot be excluded that antibodies to HLA Class I, in addition to their possible role in trapping neutrophils through their Fc receptors and activating the pulmonary endothelium, can also prime and/or activate neutrophils. Currently, there are only case reports from neutrophil (ie, granulocyte) transfusions indicating that HLA antibodies are capable of interacting with neutrophils directly (see below), and this issue awaits further experimental clarification.

In 2001, antibodies to HLA Class II were reported to be associated with TRALI in a series of 11 patients.[75] Although there is growing epidemiologic evidence for TRALI induction by HLA Class II antibodies, the biologic mechanism by which these antibodies induce TRALI remains to be elucidated. Corresponding HLA Class II antigens are not expressed on resting human neutrophils or endothelial cells, although they may be expressed on both cell types upon stimulation.[76] However, expression of HLA Class II antigens was not present on the vascular endothelium of pulmonary capillaries or intravascular neutrophils in a patient who experienced fatal TRALI.[65] Binding of HLA Class II antibodies to monocytes with subsequent release of cytokines and neutrophil activation has been suggested to constitute an alternate pathway of TRALI induction.[66] Monocytes expressing the cognate HLA Class II antigen are probably primed by the antibodies, and interaction of the primed monocytes with activated endothelial cells subsequently induces the monocytes to release neutrophil-attracting and -stimulating mediators.[67]

Further evidence is required, especially regarding the questions of whether local monocytes are able to produce sufficient amounts of cytokines and whether this multistep pathway is fast enough to explain the rapid onset of TRALI. Although HLA Class II has been found on alveolar macrophages, and although anti-HLA Class II binding to these cells may induce the release of cytokines and the subsequent activation of neutrophils and/or endothelial cells, it seems unlikely that antibodies have access to these macrophages through an intact endothelial/epithelial barrier. Still, once the barrier has been destroyed, such a reaction may exacerbate TRALI, but none of these hypotheses has yet been investigated.

Finally, antibodies to HNA and HLA could be surrogates for antibodies to—for example—monocytes. Alloantibodies to these or other cells might explain some apparently antibody-negative cases.

Bioactive Lipids

Blood components may accumulate intermediate metabolic products such as bioactive lipids during storage. These substances are breakdown products of membrane lipids, including lysophosphatidylcholines (C16, C18 lyso-PAF), and they act on neutrophils through the cells' PAF receptors in order to prime the respiratory burst reaction.[61] Because these neutrophil-priming agents do not develop in stored acellular plasma, their generation is dependent on the presence of blood cells. In a series of TRALI patients, it has been demonstrated that posttransfusion sera from these patients contained significantly more neutrophil-priming activity than did controls.[6] In addition, bioactive lipids have been reported to induce TRALI after the transfusion of stored autologous blood.[77] These findings were further investigated in an ex-vivo rat lung model of TRALI. Pretreatment of rats with LPS and exposure of the isolated lungs to plasma obtained from stored, but not from fresh, RBCs induced TRALI because of the presence of neutrophil-priming lipids.[60] Comparable results were obtained with plasma from stored, but again not from fresh, platelet concentrates.[19]

CD40-Ligand

Another neutrophil-priming breakdown product, which does not belong to the family of lipids, was identified recently as CD40-ligand (CD40L). CD40L is a primarily platelet-derived proinflammatory mediator found in cell-associated and soluble (sCD40L) forms. It has been described to be present in platelet concentrates where it accumulates during storage.[78] Its concentration in transfused platelet concentrates that were involved in TRALI cases was significantly higher than in the control units.[79]

CD40L binds to CD40, which is present on the surface of monocytes, macrophages, and neutrophils. The binding of CD40L to neutrophils can induce neutrophil priming. In vitro, human microvascular endothelial cells (HMVECs) preincubated with LPS experienced severe damage when sCD40L-primed neutrophils were added, whereas unprimed neutrophils did not induce HMVEC damage.[79] Accordingly, CD40L constitutes a possible cofactor in TRALI.

Inverse TRALI

In most cases of TRALI, antibodies or neutrophil-priming agents present in the blood component are the cause of the pulmonary reaction. However, it should not go unmentioned that TRALI has also been described in alloimmunized patients receiving components that contain neutrophils. This situation has particular relevance to patients receiving neutrophil transfusions.[80,81] In one of the case reports, a recipient was immunized against HLA-A2, and the transfused neutrophils were HLA-A2 positive.[81] It should be stated that these HLA antibodies interacted directly with the transfused cells because, as alloantibodies, these antibodies will not bind to autologous endothelial cells to commence the pathologic cascade recently reported.[16] Rather, these antibodies bind to the cognate alloantigen on the surface of the transfused leukocytes where they induce priming, sequestration within the lungs, and development of TRALI. In-vivo studies performed with 111-indium-labeled neutrophils that have been transfused in patients with neutrophil agglutinins point in the same direction, because these cells were abnormally sequestered in the lungs.[82] Most likely, after antibody-dependent neutrophil priming, "stiff" neutrophils were trapped in the pulmonary capillaries. Viable neutrophils may also be present in other cellular nonleukocyte-reduced blood components; Popovsky and Moore reported that up to 6% of all TRALI cases resulted from antibodies present in the recipient.[3] However, with the increasing use of leukocyte-reduced components, antibody binding to contaminating leukocytes in platelet and erythrocyte concentrates will become less important. However, it will remain of particular interest to patients receiving granulocyte transfusions.

Summary

TRALI shares a common pathophysiology with ALI, but the difference is that, in TRALI, the lung injury is connected to a transfusion event in a temporal and causative manner. Transfusion causes or contributes to neutrophil activation, a process that is central to the pathogenesis of TRALI. Trapped in the pulmonary capillaries, activated neutrophils release their microbicidal arsenal and injure the pulmonary endothelium, resulting in capillary leak and neutrophil transmigration. There is clear epidemiologic and experimental evidence that, in many TRALI cases, the presence of donor-derived leukocyte-reactive antibodies (ie, antibodies directed against HLA and HNA) in the blood component is the causative transfusion-related factor. Nonimmune triggers such as bioactive lipids in stored blood components have been suggested as additional potential inducers of TRALI. Neutrophil preactivation resulting from constitutive and comorbidity-related factors can modulate the patient's susceptibility to TRALI. Further improvement in understanding the pathophysiology of TRALI and its inducers will help to develop potent preventive measures.

References

1. Barnard RD. Indiscriminate transfusion: A critique of case reports illustrating hypersensitivity reactions. N Y State J Med 1951;51:2399-402.
2. Popovsky MA, Abel MD, Moore SB. Transfusion-related acute lung injury associated with passive transfer of antileukocyte antibodies. Am Rev Respir Dis 1983;128:185-9.
3. Popovsky MA, Moore SB. Diagnostic and pathogenetic considerations in transfusion-related acute lung injury. Transfusion 1985;25:573-7.
4. Wolf CF, Canale VC. Fatal pulmonary hypersensitivity reaction to HLA incompatible blood transfusion: Report of a case and review of the literature. Transfusion 1976;16:135-40.
5. Kernoff PB, Durrant IJ, Rizza CR, Wright FW. Severe allergic pulmonary oedema after plasma transfusion. Br J Haematol 1972;23:777-81.
6. Silliman CC, Paterson AJ, Dickey WO, et al. The association of biologically active lipids with the development of transfusion-related acute lung injury: A retrospective study. Transfusion 1997;37:719-26.
7. Flury R, Reutter F. Lethal anaphylactic shock during the transfusion of a thrombocyte concentrate. Schweiz Med Wochenschr 1966;96:918-20.

8. Felbo M, Jensen KG. Death in childbirth following transfusion of leukocyte-in-compatible blood. Acta Haematol 1962;27:113-19.

9. Dry SM, Bechard KM, Milford EL, et al. The pathology of transfusion-related acute lung injury. Am J Clin Pathol 1999;112:216-21.

10. Brittingham TE. Immunologic studies on leukocytes. Vox Sang 1957;2:242-8.

11. Dooren MC, Ouwehand WH, Verhoeven AJ, et al. Adult respiratory distress syndrome after experimental intravenous gamma-globulin concentrate and monocyte-reactive IgG antibodies. Lancet 1998;352:1601-2.

12. Flesch BK, Neppert J. Transfusion-related acute lung injury caused by human leucocyte antigen class II antibody. Br J Haematol 2002;116:673-6.

13. Win N, Massey E, Lucas G, et al. Ninety-six suspected transfusion-related acute lung injury cases: Investigation, findings and clinical outcome. Hematology 2007;12:461-9.

14. Seeger W, Schneider U, Kreusler B, et al. Reproduction of transfusion-related acute lung injury in an ex vivo lung model. Blood 1990;76:1438-44.

15. Sachs UJ, Hattar K, Weissmann N, et al. Antibody-induced neutrophil activation as a trigger for transfusion-related acute lung injury in an ex vivo rat lung model. Blood 2006;107:1217-19.

16. Looney MR, Su X, Van Ziffle JA, et al. Neutrophils and their Fc gamma receptors are essential in a mouse model of transfusion-related acute lung injury. J Clin Invest 2006;116:1615-23.

17. Silliman CC, Ambruso DR, Boshkov LK. Transfusion-related acute lung injury. Blood 2005;105:2266-73.

18. Bux J, Sachs UJ. The pathogenesis of transfusion-related acute lung injury (TRALI). Br J Haematol 2007;136:788-99.

19. Silliman CC, Bjornsen AJ, Wyman TH, et al. Plasma and lipids from stored platelets cause acute lung injury in an animal model. Transfusion 2003;43: 633-40.

20. Gebb SA, Graham JA, Hanger CC, et al. Sites of leukocyte sequestration in the pulmonary microcirculation. J Appl Physiol 1995;79:493-7.

21. Doerschuk CM. Neutrophil rheology and transit through capillaries and sinusoids. Am J Respir Crit Care Med 1999;159:1693-5.

22. Peters AM. Just how big is the pulmonary granulocyte pool? Clin Sci (Lond) 1998;94:7-19.

23. Loosli CG, Baker RF. Acute experimental pneumococcal (type I) pneumonia in the mouse: The migration of leucocytes from the pulmonary capillaries into the alveolar space as revealed by the electron microscope. Trans Am Clin Climatol Assoc 1962;74:15-28.

24. Downey GP, Worthen GS, Henson PM, Hyde DM. Neutrophil sequestration and migration in localized pulmonary inflammation: Capillary localization and migration across the interalveolar septum. Am Rev Respir Dis 1993;147:168-76.

25. Lee WL, Downey GP. Neutrophil activation and acute lung injury. Curr Opin Crit Care 2001;7:1-7.

26. Burns AR, Smith CW, Walker DC. Unique structural features that influence neutrophil emigration into the lung. Physiol Rev 2003;83:309-36.

27. Reutershan J, Ley K. Bench-to-bedside review: Acute respiratory distress syndrome—how neutrophils migrate into the lung. Crit Care 2004;8:453-61.

28. Issekutz AC, Rowter D, Springer TA. Role of ICAM-1 and ICAM-2 and alternate CD11/CD18 ligands in neutrophil transendothelial migration. J Leukoc Biol 1999;65:117-26.

29. Chavakis T, Preissner KT, Santoso S. Leukocyte transendothelial migration: JAMs add new pieces to the puzzle. Thromb Haemost 2003;89:13-17.

30. Ware LB, Matthay MA. Clinical practice: Acute pulmonary edema. N Engl J Med 2005;353:2788-96.

31. Guthrie LA, McPhail LC, Henson PM, Johnston RB Jr. Priming of neutrophils for enhanced release of oxygen metabolites by bacterial lipopolysaccharide: Evidence for increased activity of the superoxide-producing enzyme. J Exp Med 1984;160:1656-71.

32. Silliman CC, Boshkov LK, Mehdizadehkashi Z, et al. Transfusion-related acute lung injury: Epidemiology and a prospective analysis of etiologic factors. Blood 2003;101:454-62.

33. Holness L, Knippen MA, Simmons L, Lachenbruch PA. Fatalities caused by TRALI. Transfus Med Rev 2004;18:184-8.

34. Krause PJ, Maderazo EG, Bannon P, et al. Neutrophil heterogeneity in patients with blunt trauma. J Lab Clin Med 1988;112:208-15.

35. Kawahito K, Kobayashi E, Ohmori M, et al. Enhanced responsiveness of circulatory neutrophils after cardiopulmonary bypass: Increased aggregability and superoxide producing capacity. Artif Organs 2000;24:37-42.

36. Bass DA, Olbrantz P, Szejda P, et al. Subpopulations of neutrophils with increased oxidative product formation in blood of patients with infection. J Immunol 1986;136:860-6.

37. Vercellotti GM, Yin HQ, Gustafson KS, et al. Platelet-activating factor primes neutrophil responses to agonists: Role in promoting neutrophil-mediated endothelial damage. Blood 1988;71:1100-7.

38. Berkow RL, Wang D, Larrick JW, et al. Enhancement of neutrophil superoxide production by preincubation with recombinant human tumor necrosis factor. J Immunol 1987;139:3783-91.

39. Daniels RH, Finnen MJ, Hill ME, Lackie JM. Recombinant human monocyte IL-8 primes NADPH-oxidase and phospholipase A2 activation in human neutrophils. Immunology 1992;75:157-63.

40. Fleischmann J, Golde DW, Weisbart RH, Gasson JC. Granulocyte-macrophage colony-stimulating factor enhances phagocytosis of bacteria by human neutrophils. Blood 1986;68:708-11.

41. Tennenberg SD, Fey DE, Lieser MJ. Oxidative priming of neutrophils by interferon-gamma. J Leukoc Biol 1993;53:301-8.

42. Busse WW, Vrtis RF, Steiner R, Dick EC. In vitro incubation with influenza virus primes human polymorphonuclear leukocyte generation of superoxide. Am J Respir Cell Mol Biol 1991;4:347-54.

43. Worthen GS, Schwab B III, Elson EL, Downey GP. Mechanics of stimulated neutrophils: Cell stiffening induces retention in capillaries. Science 1989;245:183-6.

44. Waddell TK, Fialkow L, Chan CK, et al. Potentiation of the oxidative burst of human neutrophils: A signaling role for L-selectin. J Biol Chem 1994;269:18485-91.

45. Liles WC, Ledbetter JA, Waltersdorph AW, Klebanoff SJ. Cross-linking of CD18 primes human neutrophils for activation of the respiratory burst in response to specific stimuli: Implications for adhesion-dependent physiological responses in neutrophils. J Leukoc Biol 1995;58:690-7.

46. Berton G, Laudanna C, Sorio C, Rossi F. Generation of signals activating neutrophil functions by leukocyte integrins: LFA-1 and gp150/95, but not CR3, are able to stimulate the respiratory burst of human neutrophils. J Cell Biol 1992;116:1007-17.

47. Crockett-Torabi E, Sulenbarger B, Smith CW, Fantone JC. Activation of human neutrophils through L-selectin and Mac-1 molecules. J Immunol 1995;154: 2291-302.

48. Sachs UJ, Chavakis T, Fung L, et al. Human alloantibody anti-Mart interferes with Mac-1-dependent leukocyte adhesion. Blood 2004;104:727-34.

49. Kopko PM, Curtis BR, Kelher M, et al. Merging the pathogenesis of transfusion-related acute lung injury: The priming activity of the 5b (HNA-3) antibody (abstract). Transfusion 2004;44:22A.

50. Silliman CC, Curtis BR, Kopko PM, et al. Donor antibodies to HNA-3a implicated in TRALI reactions prime neutrophils and cause PMN-mediated damage to human pulmonary microvascular endothelial cells in a two-event, in vitro model. Blood 2006;109:1752-5.

51. Methods for detection of granulocyte antibodies. In: McCullough J, Press C, Clay M, Kline W, eds. Granulocyte serology: A clinical and laboratory guide. 1st ed. Chicago: American Society of Clinical Pathologists, 1988:12-14.

52. Spertini O, Luscinskas FW, Kansas GS, et al. Leukocyte adhesion molecule-1 (LAM-1, L-selectin) interacts with an inducible endothelial cell ligand to support leukocyte adhesion. J Immunol 1991;147:2565-73.

53. Gerritsen ME, Bloor CM. Endothelial cell gene expression in response to injury. FASEB J 1993;7:523-32.

54. Klein CL, Bittinger F, Skarke CC, et al. Effects of cytokines on the expression of cell adhesion molecules by cultured human omental mesothelial cells. Pathobiology 1995;63:204-12.

55. Scholz D, Devaux B, Hirche A, et al. Expression of adhesion molecules is specific and time-dependent in cytokine-stimulated endothelial cells in culture. Cell Tissue Res 1996;284:415-23.

56. Yamaguchi K, Nishio K, Sato N, et al. Leukocyte kinetics in the pulmonary microcirculation: Observations using real-time confocal luminescence microscopy coupled with high-speed video analysis. Lab Invest 1997;76:809-22.

57. Kubo H, Doyle NA, Graham L, et al. L- and P-selectin and CD11/CD18 in intracapillary neutrophil sequestration in rabbit lungs. Am J Respir Crit Care Med 1999;159:267-74.

58. Zarbock A, Singbartl K, Ley K. Complete reversal of acid-induced acute lung injury by blocking of platelet-neutrophil aggregation. J Clin Invest 2006;116: 3211-19.

59. Williams MA, Solomkin JS. Integrin-mediated signaling in human neutrophil functioning. J Leukoc Biol 1999;65:725-36.

60. Silliman CC, Voelkel NF, Allard JD, et al. Plasma and lipids from stored packed red blood cells cause acute lung injury in an animal model. J Clin Invest 1998; 101:1458-67.

61. Silliman CC, Clay KL, Thurman GW, et al. Partial characterization of lipids that develop during the routine storage of blood and prime the neutrophil NADPH oxidase. J Lab Clin Med 1994;124:684-94.

62. Dykes A, Smallwood D, Kotsimbos T, Street A. Transfusion-related acute lung injury (TRALI) in a patient with a single lung transplant. Br J Haematol 2000;109:674-6.

63. Mulligan MS, Varani J, Warren JS, et al. Roles of beta 2 integrins of rat neutrophils in complement- and oxygen radical-mediated acute inflammatory injury. J Immunol 1992;148:1847-57.

64. Rattan V, Sultana C, Shen Y, Kalra VK. Oxidant stress-induced transendothelial migration of monocytes is linked to phosphorylation of PECAM-1. Am J Physiol 1997;273:E453-61.

65. Kao GS, Wood IG, Dorfman DM, et al. Investigations into the role of anti-HLA class II antibodies in TRALI. Transfusion 2003;43:185-91.

66. Kopko PM, Paglieroni TG, Popovsky MA, et al. TRALI: Correlation of antigen-antibody and monocyte activation in donor-recipient pairs. Transfusion 2003; 43:177-84.

67. Nishimura M, Hashimoto S, Takanashi M, et al. Role of anti-human leucocyte antigen class II alloantibody and monocytes in development of transfusion-related acute lung injury. Transfus Med 2007;17:129-34.

68. Taylor FB, Chang AC, Peer G, et al. Active site inhibited factor VIIa (DEGR VIIa) attenuates the coagulant and interleukin-6 and -8, but not tumor necrosis factor, responses of the baboon to LD_{100} Escherichia coli. Blood 1998;91: 1609-15.

69. Hammerschmidt DE, Weaver LJ, Hudson LD, et al. Association of complement activation and elevated plasma-C5a with adult respiratory distress syndrome: Pathophysiological relevance and possible prognostic value. Lancet 1980;1: 947-9.

70. Yomtovian R, Kline W, Press C, et al. Severe pulmonary hypersensitivity associated with passive transfusion of a neutrophil-specific antibody. Lancet 1984;1: 244-6.

71. Nordhagen R, Conradi M, Dromtorp SM. Pulmonary reaction associated with transfusion of plasma containing anti-5b. Vox Sang 1986;51:102-7.

72. Bux J, Becker F, Seeger W, et al. Transfusion-related acute lung injury due to HLA-A2-specific antibodies in recipient and NB1-specific antibodies in donor blood. Br J Haematol 1996;93:707-13.

73. Leach M, Vora AJ, Jones DA, Lucas G. Transfusion-related acute lung injury (TRALI) following autologous stem cell transplant for relapsed acute myeloid leukaemia: A case report and review of the literature. Transfus Med 1998;8: 333-7.

74. Bux J. Transfusion-related acute lung injury (TRALI): A serious adverse event of blood transfusion. Vox Sang 2005;89:1-10.

75. Kopko PM, Popovsky MA, MacKenzie MR, et al. HLA class II antibodies in transfusion-related acute lung injury. Transfusion 2001;41:1244-8.

76. Gosselin EJ, Wardwell K, Rigby WF, Guyre PM. Induction of MHC class II on human polymorphonuclear neutrophils by granulocyte/macrophage colony-stimulating factor, IFN-gamma, and IL-3. J Immunol 1993;151:1482-90.

77. Covin RB, Ambruso DR, England KM, et al. Hypotension and acute pulmonary insufficiency following transfusion of autologous red blood cells during surgery: A case report and review of the literature. Transfus Med 2004;14:375-83.

78. Phipps RP, Kaufman J, Blumberg N. Platelet-derived CD154 (CD40 ligand) and febrile responses to transfusion. Lancet 2001;357:2023-4.

79. Khan SY, Kelher MR, Heal JM, et al. Soluble CD40 ligand accumulates in stored blood components, primes neutrophils through CD40, and is a potential cofactor in the development of transfusion-related acute lung injury. Blood 2006;108:2455-62.

80. O'Connor JC, Strauss RG, Goeken NE, Knox LB. A near-fatal reaction during granulocyte transfusion of a neonate. Transfusion 1988;28:173-6.

81. Sachs UJ, Bux J. TRALI after the transfusion of cross-match-positive granulocytes. Transfusion 2003;43:1683-6.

82. McCullough J, Clay M, Hurd D, et al. Effect of leukocyte antibodies and HLA matching on the intravascular recovery, survival, and tissue localization of 111-indium granulocytes. Blood 1986;67:522-8.

In: Kleinman S, Popovsky MA, eds.
TRALI: Mechanisms, Management, and Prevention
Bethesda, MD: AABB Press, 2008

4

Donor Management and Laboratory Investigation of Suspected TRALI

RICHARD J. BENJAMIN, MD, PhD, FRCPath, AND
ANNE F. EDER, MD, PhD

THE CANADIAN CONSENSUS CONFERENCE panel and a National Heart, Lung, and Blood Institute (NHLBI) working group define transfusion-related acute lung injury (TRALI) as a clinical syndrome consisting of new acute lung injury (ALI) occurring within 6 hours of transfusion in the absence of preexisting ALI.[1,2] TRALI is further differentiated from "possible TRALI" (suspected TRALI occurring in the presence of other possible causes of ALI) and fluid overload (transfusion-associated circulatory overload, or TACO).[1,3] Because the diagnosis of

Richard J. Benjamin, MD, PhD, FRCPath, Chief Medical Officer, and Anne F. Eder, MD, PhD, Executive Medical Officer, Biomedical Services, American Red Cross Blood Services, National Headquarters, Washington, District of Columbia

TRALI is based on clinical findings, the definitions make no assumptions about the etiology of the reaction and do not rely on the laboratory investigation of the associated donors. Nonetheless, the consensus panel recognized the importance of laboratory investigation in order to determine a donor's continued eligibility to donate.

Blood collection facilities are obligated by US federal law to investigate adverse reactions related to transfusion, including TRALI, and the Food and Drug Administration (FDA) Blood Products Advisory Committee (BPAC) has recommended that donors implicated in multiple cases of TRALI be identified and deferred.[4] Blood collectors should question 1) whether the donors associated with a proven case of TRALI may cause a reaction in other recipients and 2) which specific interventions are appropriate to mitigate risk. Such logic demands that blood centers formally and extensively investigate donors of blood components that are thought to cause TRALI and that they defer or redirect donors who have increased risk of causing reactions in future recipients. In practice, this obligation is difficult to fulfill and blood centers are frequently faced with making individualized decisions about the extent of investigations, including which cases to investigate, whether to perform testing on all or selected donors, which tests to perform, and how to manage the results from these investigations. This chapter aims to define the issues involved in managing donors in TRALI cases and suggests a strategy going forward according to a review of the literature, current US and international practice, and expert opinion.

The Canadian Consensus Conference Recommendations for Donor Management

The Canadian Consensus Conference panel recognized that preventing future donation by blood donors associated with TRALI cases may reduce the risk among transfused patients. However, after being presented with different approaches by conference speakers, the panel was not able to reach consensus on a set of recommendations for donor management. Instead, the panel attempted to delineate the issues and created formal definitions of donor involvement to clarify future discussions: a donor is *associated* with TRALI if one of his or her blood components was transfused during the 6 hours preceding the first clinical manifestation of TRALI, and a donor is *implicated* if found to have detectable antibodies to a human neutrophil antigen (HNA) or Class I or II HLA present on the recipient's leukocytes.[1]

The panel considered and rejected a uniform approach that would defer all donors associated with TRALI reactions from future donation or would restrict them to whole blood donation, with Washed Red Blood Cells (RBCs) as the only allowable transfusable component from their donations. The panel also discussed tracking associated donors by electronically "flagging" any future donation so that they could be deferred if again associated with TRALI in a subsequent transfusion. This approach, however, was not endorsed because some members of the panel raised the ethical argument that such action may fail to avoid a future TRALI reaction and may complicate the informed consent process—if jurisdictions consider a "flagged" donor as a reasonable risk that should be disclosed to the patient. Ultimately, the panel favored a targeted approach, with laboratory investigation of *associated* donors in confirmed TRALI. Deferral of only the donors who were implicated was viewed as likely to prevent TRALI in future recipients and would avoid the unnecessary deferral of donors who posed little or no risk. The panel could not reach consensus on the management of donors associated with "possible TRALI" cases and left the decision to investigate and/or to defer to the blood collecting facilities.

The algorithm for donor investigation recommended by the consensus panel is based first on a formal and complete investigation of each case to distinguish among TRALI, possible TRALI, and TACO, followed by an investigation of all the donors in cases that have a clear diagnosis of TRALI. The investigation would include a sample that is from each donor and is screened for HLA and HNA antibodies, plus a recipient sample that could be used for HLA- or HNA-antigen testing, if indicated. If the antibody screen demonstrates the presence of reactivity in one or more donor samples, the specificity of the antibodies should be identified, and the recipient sample should be HLA- and HNA-typed to determine a match. Alternatively, a direct crossmatch test could be performed to determine if the donor's antibodies recognize the recipient's leukocytes. The sample for testing may be obtained from the blood component residual volume, from a co-component from the same donation, or, more frequently, from another blood sample obtained from the donor.

The panel noted the expense and logistical issues around conducting complete TRALI donor investigations and discussed whether selective or sequential donor testing is feasible.

A selective approach limits testing to certain donors (eg, previously pregnant or transfused), whereas a sequential approach may prioritize the order in which donors are tested and may halt further testing if an antibody-positive donor is identified. For example, donors whose components were administered closest to the onset of TRALI might be tested first; or donors of plasma, platelets, cryoprecipitated AHF, and red cells might be tested in that order; or multiparous female donors, other female donors, and then male donors might be tested. Although accepting that a selective or sequential approach is feasible, the panel emphasized that an approach should be chosen regardless of the number of donors associated with a given reaction. Because the investigation is confined to the components transfused within 6 hours preceding the onset of TRALI, the number of donors in any given case is usually manageable, even when all the associated donors must be tested. The panel noted that some TRALI reactions are caused by recipient leukocyte antibodies reacting with donor leukocytes; however, they considered the related laboratory investigation to be unnecessary in routine practice because most components are leukocyte reduced. Likewise, investigation for neutrophil priming activity was not recommended as part of a routine TRALI case investigation.[1]

Assuming a protocol of full investigation of all donors, the panel recommended that donors implicated in TRALI should be either permanently deferred from whole blood and apheresis platelet and plasma donation or allowed to donate if the only components produced from the donation were washed or (frozen) deglycerolized RBCs and plasma for fractionation. These policy recommendations were based on the limited look-back investigations that were available at that time documenting instances in which donors with antibodies were implicated in TRALI reactions in multiple recipients,[5,6] and on an overall precautionary approach to protecting transfusion recipients, recognizing that some safe donors might be inadvertently deferred by this policy.

Furthermore, the panel recognized that donor investigations might not be complete because of difficulty in obtaining suitable donor and recipient specimens. Blood centers may be left to make donor deferral decisions without sufficient information to determine whether a donor was implicated, associated, or excluded by the investigation. Furthermore, donors with antibodies that failed to match with any of the patient's antigens (noncognate antibodies) may be identified. At that time, no consensus was reached with respect to their future eligibility to donate. However, the panel stated that there was sufficient evidence to recommend the indefinite deferral of donors bearing specific HNA antibodies (but not nonspecific HNA antibodies), particularly HNA-3a antibodies, that have been repeatedly implicated in TRALI reactions.[5] Donors with negative tests for HLA and/or HNA antibodies, however, may continue to donate whether or not the TRALI case investigation identified an implicated donor because there is no evidence that such antibody-negative, TRALI-associated donors pose an additional risk to future transfusion recipients.

Deferral: Recommendations and Variations

The Rationale for Donor Deferral

The etiology of TRALI likely involves the activation of granulocytes that target and destroy the pulmonary capillary/alveolar interface, leading to an extravasation of protein-rich fluid into the alveolar space.[7] (See Chapter 3.) The patient's susceptibility to these events may be influenced by multiple factors, including his or her underlying condition (eg, sepsis, shock, burns, infection), substances (eg, bioactive response mediators) that accumulate with storage in blood components, or the presence of specific alloreactive antibodies in the donated components that target recipient leukocytes, endothelium, or both.[8] Two or more of these factors are likely necessary to trigger TRALI. Blood centers, however, can directly manage only donor risk, whereas hospital transfusion services and the attending clinicians are better able to control the risks associated with transfusion practice. It seems likely that focused interventions for donor, component, and recipient factors will be required to effectively mitigate all risks for TRALI. For the present, the identification and deferral of at-risk donors are the only active preventive measures in common practice; even then, the transfusion community is uncertain about the optimum management strategy.

AABB Recommendations

The uncertainty described above is evidenced by the relevant AABB standard (Standard 5.4.2.1): "Donors implicated in a TRALI event or associated with multiple events of TRALI shall be evaluated regarding their continued eligibility to donate."[9(p21)] In this instance, "implicated" is defined according to the consensus panel definition—that is, involving a component that was transfused within 6 hours of a proven TRALI reaction and that has been shown to contain an HLA or HNA antibody toward an antigen that is expressed by the recipient.[10] The standard allows for broad interpretation because neither the extent of investigation required nor the consequences for the implicated donor is specified.

In 2006, the AABB recommended in an *Association Bulletin* that "blood collecting facilities should implement interventions to minimize the preparation of high plasma-volume components from donors known to be leukocyte-alloimmunized or at increased risk of leukocyte alloimmunization."[11] Although it is only a broad recommendation, blood centers are encouraged to act to prevent transfusion of high plasma-volume products from donors with alloantibodies (HLA or HNA), thus suggesting that if antibodies are detected, donors should be either indefinitely deferred or redirected to donate low plasma-volume products for transfusion.

Variations in Practice

The AABB standard and *Association Bulletin* are the only guidance available to the blood community for the management of donors associated with TRALI (and no regulatory guidance exists), even though TRALI is recognized as the most frequent life-threatening complication related to transfusion.[12] Not surprisingly, substantial variability in practice is documented in a recent survey. Performed in July 2006[13] by the AABB (45% of blood centers and 66% of hospital-based blood collectors reporting), this survey documents that, in practice, the diagnosis of TRALI is frequently based on the results of both clinical and laboratory investigations, contrary to the consensus panel recommendations that define TRALI as a clinical diagnosis. Moreover, although "almost all" US blood collectors test for both HLA Class I and II antibodies in donors associated with TRALI reactions, 1) HNA testing is performed much less frequently (51% of blood centers and 37% of hospital-based collectors reporting), 2) recipient specimens for HLA and HNA typing are rarely obtained (68% to 73% of blood collectors reported that recipient samples were available in <25% of TRALI investigations), and 3) donors are frequently selectively tested according to gender, history of transfusion or pregnancy, or proximity of the transfusion to the onset of symptoms. Finally, although there is general agreement among the responding institutions that donors implicated in TRALI should be deferred from future donation, many respondents tailor their case investigations and deferral policies on a case-by-case basis. The authors of the survey conclude that some of this variation may be the result of incomplete knowledge and uncertainty regarding TRALI, and they argue for increased education of transfusion medicine practitioners as one solution to determining a consensus approach to donor management in TRALI.

Similar variation in practice has been documented in an international survey that included questions about the management of donors associated with, or implicated in, cases of TRALI (Table 4-1). Respondents from 14 nations summarized their understanding of TRALI donor management in their own countries, where, in each case, there are no nationally determined guidelines set by regulatory authorities.[4] The situation where consensus was approached most nearly was found in the case of a donor implicated in a proven case of TRALI, where 11 of 14 responding countries would permanently defer the donor from all donation, whereas in two countries, donors would be deferred only from donating Fresh Frozen Plasma (FFP) and/or platelets for transfusion. In the United States, 95% of the blood centers but only 44% of the hospital blood collectors would permanently defer donors from all donation in this same scenario.

Consensus was poor for donors associated with, but not implicated in, a given case of TRALI: 6 of 14 country respondents would permanently defer these donors, and the others would selectively defer donors from donating high plasma-volume components for transfusion (4 countries), track donors and defer them if a donor is associated with a second TRALI case (2 countries), or selectively defer on the basis of the specificity of the antibody detected (2 countries). In the United States, 39% of the blood centers and 1.4% of the hospital blood collectors would defer the donors in this setting.

Finally, if investigation of a TRALI case failed to detect antibodies in a given donor plasma, respondents from 2 countries would still permanently defer the donor, whereas the others might reinstate the donor to full donation (6 countries), selectively defer the donor from donating high plasma-volume components for transfusion (2 countries), track and defer if associated with a second case of TRALI, or defer if there were only one donor involved in the TRALI case. In the United States, 34% of the blood centers and 5.5% of the hospital blood col-

Table 4-1. International Variability in the Management of Donors Associated with TRALI Reactions*

	Policy if Donor Is Implicated?	Policy if Antibodies Are Present but Not Reactive with Patient Cells?	Policy if No Antibodies Are Detected?
Brazil	Practice is to permanently defer.	Practice is to permanently defer.	Practice is to permanently defer.
Denmark	Practice is to not use FFP. If implicated in two or more cases, defer.	Practice is to not use FFP. If implicated in two or more cases, defer.	Practice is to not use FFP. If implicated in two or more cases, defer.
Finland	Practice is to permanently defer.	If reliable TRALI diagnosis, practice is to permanently defer.	If reliable TRALI diagnosis, practice is to permanently defer.
Germany	Practice is to not use FFP or Platelets for transfusion.	Practice is to not use FFP or Platelets for transfusion.	Practice is to not use FFP or Platelets if donor has a history of pregnancy or transfusion.
Ireland	Practice is to permanently defer.	If reliable TRALI diagnosis, investigate female donors and males with transfusion history. Practice is to permanently defer.	Donors are reinstated to donate again.
Japan	Practice is to not use any products for transfusion.	Practice is to not use any products for transfusion.	No action is taken.

(Continued)

Table 4-1. International Variability in the Management of Donors Associated with TRALI Reactions* (Continued)

	Policy if Donor Is Implicated?	Policy if Antibodies Are Present but Not Reactive with Patient Cells?	Policy if No Antibodies Are Detected?
The Netherlands	Practice is to permanently defer.	Practice is to continue donation and track. If implicated in two or more cases, defer.	Practice is to continue donation and track. If implicated in two or more cases, defer.
New Zealand	Practice is to permanently defer.	Practice is to permanently defer.	Donors are reinstated to donate again.
Norway	Practice is to permanently defer.	Defer if only one donor involved; otherwise continue donation and track. If implicated in two or more cases, defer.	Defer if only one donor involved; otherwise, continue donation and track. If implicated in two or more cases, defer.
Poland	Practice is to permanently defer.	Defer if HLA-A2, HNA-3a, or HNA nonspecific antibodies.	Temporarily defer, assess adequacy of investigation, and perform crossmatch, if possible.

Spain	Practice is to permanently defer.	If HNA or HLA Class II antibodies, permanently defer. If HLA Class I antibodies, continue to donate low plasma-volume components.	No action is taken.
Switzerland	Practice is to permanently defer.	Practice is to permanently defer if strongly reactive. Donors with weak antibodies may donate RBCs and plasma for fractionation.	No action is taken.
United Kingdom	Practice is to permanently defer.	Donors may donate whole blood; however, platelets and plasma are not manufactured.	Donors may continue to donate but are tracked for future involvement in TRALI.
United States	95% of donor centers would defer, and 44% of hospital collectors would defer.	If recipient type does not match, 39% and 1.4% of donor centers and hospital collectors would defer.	If single donor involved, 34% and 5.5% of donor centers and hospital collectors would defer. If multiple donors, no deferral.
US FDA	No FDA guidance on donor management. BPAC recommended deferral of donors implicated in multiple cases of TRALI.	No FDA guidance on donor management.	No FDA guidance on donor management.

*Questions related to the management of donors involved in a case of TRALI. Data derived from Wendel et al.[4]
FFP = Fresh Frozen Plasma; HNA = human neutrophil antigen; RBCs = Red Blood Cells; FDA = Food and Drug Administration; BPAC = Blood Products Advisory Committee.

lectors would permanently defer a donor from all donation if a single donor was associated with a given case, regardless of the outcome of laboratory investigations.[4,13]

These surveys highlight the wide variety of practices, both in the United States and abroad, for the management of donors of blood components involved in TRALI. In the absence of clear regulatory instruction or industry standards, blood collection centers have complete medical discretion to manage donors according to local practice. The risk of this approach is that attention may be focused on the donor as an individual and not as the potential source of a high-risk blood component. In regulatory terms, this situation may represent a failure to ensure adequate quality control in the production of components intended for transfusion.

Evidence that Donor Deferral Can Prevent the Incidence of TRALI

Is there a scientific basis on which donors associated with TRALI cases should be managed? If alloreactive antibodies directed against HLA or HNA antigens trigger TRALI, preventing transfusion of components with these antibodies should prevent TRALI. The evidence that alloreactive antibodies, in general, cause TRALI is reasonably strong but circumstantial. Many studies have shown a higher proportion of donors with alloantibodies associated with TRALI cases. Cognate recognition of recipient antigens is frequently documented, and ex-vivo and animal studies show that certain alloantibodies can trigger ALI.[8,14-17] This is particularly true for alloantibodies recognizing HNA antibodies.[18] However, Koch's postulates for disease causation have not been met, and it is worthwhile to retain a degree of skepticism about incriminating an antibody in any given case.

Recent studies have shown that 10% to 20% of females and 1% to 4% of untransfused males harbor HLA antibodies.[19-22] Although pregnancy clearly stimulates a higher prevalence of antibodies, it appears that both males and females may exhibit

HLA antibodies without known exposure to alloantigen through transfusion or pregnancy. The clinical significance of these antibodies in their ability to cause TRALI is unknown. The obvious incongruity is that leukocyte alloantibodies are common, whereas TRALI occurs in only about 1:5000 transfusions (varying from 1:400 to 1:500,000 in different studies examining various components and patient population groups).[1,23]

Many TRALI cases involve multiply transfused individuals, raising the probability that an alloantibody detected during an investigation of TRALI, even with proven cognate recognition, may occur by chance alone. A chance association is especially possible for antibodies directed against common antigens, such as HLA-A2 or HNA-3a. The properties of an antibody that determine its functional activity include not only its antigenic specificity, but also its isotype, avidity, epitope specificity, concentration, and titer, as well as the availability and activation state of effector functions at the time of antigen recognition. These functions may include Fc receptor-mediated effects (eg, antibody-dependent cellular cytotoxicity), as well as interaction with complement and its inhibitors. Cognate recognition is, therefore, necessary but not sufficient to prove causation by a given antibody, although the current definition of donors "implicated" in TRALI assumes cause and effect and directly influences donor deferral actions.[10]

Prospective randomized trials are necessary 1) to prove that deferring donors implicated in TRALI cases is efficacious in reducing the incidence of TRALI and 2) to provide supportive evidence that cognate recognition is sufficient for causation. However, it is unlikely that these studies will be performed because of both logistic and ethical considerations. In the absence of prospective studies, direct evidence that the risk from a given alloantibody might be reduced through donor deferral has been sought through retrospective look-back studies. An indirect measure of the danger of a particular antibody is the frequency with which transfusions from that donor have triggered adverse transfusion reactions in the past, which have been reported for HLA Class I and II antibodies and/or HNA antibodies in look-back studies (Table 4-2).

Table 4-2. Case Reports of Look-Back Investigations of Donors Implicated in TRALI

Investigation	Index Component	Donor Antibody Identified	Components Investigated (units)	Evaluable Patients	Reactions Identified on Look-Back Investigation	Suspected TRALI Identified on Look-Back Investigation
Nicolle et al[24]	FFP	HLA-DR4	6 RBC, 3 FFP	9	1 (hemolytic)	0
Nicolle et al[24]	FFP	HLA-A2, -A9, -DR4	7 RBC, 2 FFP	9	1	1
Kopko et al[5]	FFP	HNA-3a	63 FFP	36	15 reactions in 13 patients	2
Win et al[25]	Pooled Platelets	HNA-1a				
Win et al[25]	FFP	HNA nonspecific	16 RBC, 17 Platelet, 10 FFP issued to 43 patients			
Win et al[25]	Cryoprecipitated AHF	HLA multispecific				
Win et al[25]	Pooled Platelets	HLA multispecific		30	0	0
Win et al[25]	FFP	HLA-A2				
Win et al[25]	Pooled Platelets	HLA multispecific				

Study	Component	Antibody	Component details			
Cooling[6]	Apheresis Platelets or FFP	HLA Class I multispecific	16 Apheresis Platelet, 4 FFP	20	3	2
Fadeyi et al[26]	Apheresis Platelets	HNA-2a	39 Apheresis Platelet	32	12	0
Toy et al[27]	Apheresis Platelets	HLA Class I/II multispecific	109 Apheresis Platelet or FFP	103	4 new pulmonary infiltrates	0
Zupanska et al[28]		HLA-A24, -A29, -B7, -DR1, -DR2		8	0	0
Zupanska et al[28]		HLA-A1, -A29, -B37, -DR8, -DR13, -DR14		12	0	0

FFP = Fresh Frozen Plasma; HNA = human neutrophil antigen; RBC = Red Blood Cell.

Kopko et al[5] reported a retrospective chart review of 50 patients who received one or more plasma components donated by a female donor who was later implicated in a fatal case of TRALI. The donor was shown to harbor a "strongly positive" HNA-3a (5b) antibody that corresponds to an antigen expressed by >90% of white Americans. Of the available patient charts, 13 of 36 (36.1%) revealed a transfusion reaction after 15 transfusion episodes. Seven mild reactions were documented, including chills, dyspnea, fever, tachycardia, chest pain, rigors, nausea, vomiting, and oxygen desaturation. Eight severe reactions included respiratory failure, pulmonary edema, chest pain, acute respiratory distress syndrome, and cardiac arrest. Only seven reactions were reported to the transfusion service and only two, including the fatality, were reported to the blood center. These data highlight the following points: 1) the majority of patients receiving blood containing HNA-3a (5b) antibody apparently suffer no adverse consequence despite cognate recognition; 2) many patients may display symptoms that are less severe and nondiagnostic for TRALI; and 3) TRALI, when it occurs, is infrequently recognized or reported to the blood center.

Similarly, Fadeyi et al[26] reported a look-back investigation of an apheresis platelet donor who was identified after investigation of a transfusion reaction that consisted of chills, fever, dyspnea, and transient leucopenia. Although this case did not meet the diagnostic criteria of TRALI, investigation revealed an HNA-2a antibody directed against an antigen expressed by 95% to 97% of the general population. Look-back investigation revealed 39 transfusions that resulted in 12 transfusion reactions in 9 patients. Symptoms included chills, rigors, fever, and, on nine occasions, signs and symptoms of respiratory insufficiency. Again, these data highlight the frequency and diverse spectrum of reactions that may occur with the transfusion of HNA antibodies and that may not meet the definition of, or be recognized as, TRALI.

Cooling[6] performed look-back investigations after a fatal TRALI case on a donor who harbored high-titer HLA Class I antibodies with broad specificity (eg, >99% panel-reactive antibodies). Among recipients of apheresis platelet or plasma components, 3 of 20 (15%) patients showed evidence of respiratory insufficiency, and 2 patients had evidence of bilateral pulmonary infiltrates. These 3 cases were not recognized at the time of transfusion as suspected TRALI reactions and were not reported to the blood center.

Nicolle et al[24] described a look-back investigation on two donors implicated in TRALI. The first donor harbored an HLA-DR4 antibody, corresponding to an antigen expressed by 34% of the population in the United Kingdom. Look-back investigation on 6 units of RBCs and 3 units of plasma revealed no evidence of a TRALI-like reaction. In contrast, the second donor harbored HLA-DR4, HLA-A2, and HLA-A9 antibodies expressed in 34%, 48%, and 29% of the British population, respectively. Investigation of 7 units of RBCs and 2 units of FFP revealed an unrecognized, but documented, TRALI-like reaction after the transfusion of a unit of FFP.

In contrast, Toy et al[27] performed an investigation on an apheresis platelet and plasma donor implicated in a fatal case of TRALI who was found to harbor multiple HLA Class I and II antibodies reactive with 96% and 88% of HLA antigens, respectively. Blood from the index donor was transfused as 109 units to 103 patients. One patient developed the clinical syndrome of TRALI but was found to have diffuse alveolar hemorrhage. A total of 78 of these patients were studied in a blinded retrospective cohort study in which reactions to a look-back transfusion were compared with paired control transfusions given to the same patient. A comparison of the outcomes revealed no difference between the test and the control transfusions relative to new hypoxemia, fever, hypotension, or change in white blood cell count. After test transfusions only, 4 of 62 patients examined showed new or worse bilateral pulmonary infiltrates, and 4 showed similar new infiltrates after both test and control transfusions (suggesting fluid overload) ($p = 0.125$). No patients developed a confirmed case of TRALI, although 54 of 55 patients who had been HLA-typed expressed cognate antigens recognized by the alloantibodies. This study highlights the frequency with which HLA antibodies may be transfused to recipients expressing cognate antigens without ill effect and emphasizes the need for controlled comparisons, given the high background of untoward effects that may not be transfusion-related, in seriously ill patients.

Win et al[25] examined six cases of proven TRALI where donors were found to harbor either multispecific or specific HLA or HNA antibodies. Look-back investigation performed on 16 RBC units, 17 platelet units (5 pooled and 12 apheresis), and 10 plasma units failed to reveal evidence of a transfusion reaction in 30 evaluable patients. Zupanska et al[28] reported a similar experience performing a look-back investigation on two donors implicated in severe TRALI cases after RBC transfusion. Although these donors expressed antibodies to a wide range of HLA antigens (HLA-A24, -A29, -B7, -DR1, and -DR2, and HLA-A1, -A29, -B37, -DR8, -DR11, -DR13, and -DR14, respectively), look-back studies on 20 transfusions reported no TRALI reactions. Milder effects, such as dyspnea, were recorded but not enumerated in this report.

Taken together, the above look-back studies reveal a total of at least 36 adverse reactions in 261 patient records examined (Table 4-2); the reactions had previously been documented in the patients' records, but often without transfusion service notification. Only 5 reactions rose to the level of a suspected TRALI diagnosis. Most of the other reactions were mild to moderate, including dyspnea, fever, and chills, or there was x-ray evidence of new pulmonary infiltrates or a combination of these factors. Because many of these reactions included pulmonary symptoms, they may have been caused by transfused antibody and may have been associated with some morbidity and treatment costs. Of the reactions, 27 were linked to an HNA antibody, whereas only 9 implicated an HLA antibody. All of these reactions were associated with plasma or apheresis platelets, not with RBC transfusions. Many transfusions involving antibodies shown to be reactive with recipient cells did not result in any documented adverse reaction.

These data allow the following conclusions:
1. TRALI is rare in look-back studies of donors with known alloantibodies and previous involvement in TRALI reactions, occurring in <2% of transfusions.

2. Less severe reactions that are not diagnostic for TRALI are documented more frequently ($\approx 14\%$ of transfusions).
3. HNA antibodies are more likely to cause reactions than HLA antibodies.
4. High plasma-volume components (apheresis platelets and plasma) are usually involved.

These conclusions may be criticized on a number of levels:

1. Most studies are poorly controlled, limiting the interpretation of the data.
2. Their retrospective design may have biased the selection of the cases on which look-back investigation was performed.
3. A dangerous donor may be deferred early in his or her donation career, thus providing few prior donations on which a look-back investigation could be performed.

Nevertheless, the data provide the best available scientific basis for the deferral of donors implicated in TRALI.

Although the deferral of implicated donors has not been subjected to prospective study as a means to reduce the incidence of TRALI, it is probably not highly efficacious in preventing TRALI in the broad view. The incidence of reported TRALI continues to rise, despite the publication of AABB Standard 5.4.2.1 that requires policies to investigate donors associated with TRALI, and the practice continues to vary among transfusion services and blood centers[12] in this regard. Nevertheless, donor deferral remains a mainstay of TRALI prevention and is the only intervention that transfusion services are required to consider according to AABB standards. Ultimately, this intervention is based on the precautionary principle and the empirical logic that a donor who is implicated in a TRALI reaction is more likely to be involved again in the future.

Donor Management: The Desired State

Donor management decisions should be consistent not only within an organization but also across the transfusion medicine community, as a fundamental quality control step in the production of blood components for transfusion. Uniform decisions would also facilitate assessment of the efficacy of individual TRALI reduction policies, as national hemovigilance programs expand.[12] Consistency requires consensus and commitment to standard deferral criteria, preferentially on the basis of sound science. Major strides in this direction are being made through studies such as the REDS II program (Retrovirus Epidemiology Donor Studies) Leukocyte Antigen Prevalence Study, funded by the National Institutes of Health, that has more precisely defined the prevalence of HLA antibodies in the donor community.[20,29] Likewise, the AABB recommendation that donors harboring alloreactive leukocyte antibodies (independent of any association with a TRALI case) be prevented from donating high plasma-volume components has led to a renewed interest by manufacturers to develop high throughput, cost-effective assays for HLA antibodies. Similar high-throughput technologies to evaluate the prevalence of HNA antibodies and prospective studies to determine the clinical significance of specific alloreactive HLA and/or HNA antibodies are needed urgently.

Technology and information of this nature would lay the basis for prospectively screening all donors for alloreactive leukocyte antibodies and for determining which donors should be permanently deferred from donation, which donors should be restricted to donate low plasma-volume components for transfusion, or which donors should be permitted to donate components of all varieties.

In the absence of complete data and given the accumulating evidence that TRALI is a major threat to the safety of blood recipients,[12] the blood community should base donor management decisions on the precautionary principle that requires "... a willingness to take action in advance of scientific proof [or] evidence of the need for the proposed action on the grounds that further delay will prove ultimately most costly to society and nature, and, in the longer term, selfish and unfair to future generations."[30]

Donor Management: State of the Art Recommendations

With the frequent lack of definitive data required to make the diagnosis of TRALI and with incomplete investigation of donor and recipient antibody and antigens, donor management has been an art that has required considerable insight by blood center physicians. The AABB has not provided definitive guidance in its standards and bulletins because of the high level of uncertainty described. Instead, facilities are encouraged to have standard processes in place to investigate TRALI cases and to manage associated donors. A number of authors have suggested approaches to donor investigation and management, and useful guidelines have been published.[1,31-33] Recently, Su and Kamel[34] have developed a consistent approach at one major blood system.

The following recommendations (summarized in Table 4-3) are the authors' attempt to formulate a rational approach that is based on the available information. Several of the identified options have been recommended by other experts in the field. Although the approach does not represent current practice in any specific blood center, it is intended to provide a framework for further discussion and consensus building in the transfusion medicine community.

1. **Promote reporting.** Blood centers should promote the recognition and reporting of ALI-type reactions by transfusion services.[1,23,34]

2. **Encourage thorough investigation.** Blood centers should work closely with the reporting transfusion services to obtain sufficient clinical information in cases of ALI after transfusion in order to determine if the criteria are met for a diagnosis of TRALI or possible TRALI according to the Canadian Consensus Conference Panel and NHLBI working group definitions. The presence or absence of alloreactive antibodies in a donor, even with cognate recognition of recipient antigens, should not influence the diagnosis of TRALI.[1,23]

Table 4-3. A Suggested Framework for Managing Donors Investigated for TRALI or Possible TRALI Reactions

Clinical Diagnosis	Cognate HLA/HNA Antibody and Antigen Match	Specific HNA Antibody Detected	Single Associated Donor; No Antibody Detected	Associated with a Prior Case of TRALI or Possible TRALI; No Antibody Detected	HLA/ Nonspecific HNA Antibody Detected but No Match with Recipient Antigen	HLA/ Nonspecific HNA Antibody Detected; No Recipient Data	Donor Investigation Not Performed	Donor Investigation Fails to Reveal HLA or HNA Antibodies and More than One Associated Donor
TRALI	Indefinite deferral	Indefinite deferral	Consider indefinite deferral* or flag donor†	Indefinite deferral	Low plasma-volume components only; flag donor†	Indefinite deferral	Defer donor until investigation completed; flag donor†	No deferral; flag donor†

Possible TRALI	Indefinite deferral	Indefinite deferral	Consider indefinite deferral* or flag donor†	Indefinite deferral	Low plasma-volume components only; flag donor†	Indefinite deferral	Defer donor until investigation completed; flag donor†	No deferral; flag donor†
TRALI or possible TRALI diagnosis is equivocal or ruled out‡	Low plasma-volume components only	Indefinite deferral	No deferral	No deferral	Low plasma-volume components only	Low plasma-volume components only	No deferral	No deferral

*On the basis of the strength of the TRALI diagnosis, involvement of a high plasma-volume component, and time between transfusion and the reaction.

†A flag in the computer system or other means serves to identify, with each subsequent TRALI investigation, that the donor has been associated with TRALI or possible TRALI.

‡Donor investigation is not recommended at all in the absence of a high level of suspicion of TRALI; however, if donor testing is performed, the approach to donor management decisions in such scenarios is given.

HNA = human neutrophil antigen.

3. **Decide about laboratory testing.** Blood collection agencies should decide whether to test donors for alloreactive antibodies on the basis of the strength of the evidence for a TRALI diagnosis and the severity of the reaction, not on the number or characteristics of the associated donors. Although some authors have suggested a selective approach to investigating TRALI cases on the basis of the number of associated donors (eg, selective testing if there are more than 4 donors[34]), the Canadian Consensus Panel recommends that all of the donors in highly probable TRALI cases should be investigated.[1]

   a. Donors associated with TRALI should be investigated as extensively as possible, particularly in life-threatening or fatal cases. All associated donors should be screened for both HLA and HNA antibodies, with recipient typing or direct crossmatch performed if any donor is found to harbor alloreactive leukocyte antibodies.[34,35]

   b. Donors associated with cases of TACO should not be further investigated for alloreactive antibodies.[1]

   c. Donors associated with cases of possible TRALI should be further investigated only if there is a high level of suspicion of TRALI, as determined through consultation between the blood center and transfusion service physician. If a case of possible TRALI is investigated because the case is thought to represent TRALI, the donor management should be the same as it would be for TRALI cases.

   d. Recipient antibodies may interact with donor leukocytes to cause TRALI. However, such a finding would not lead to donor deferral and does not assist in the diagnosis of TRALI. Consequently, the authors do not recommend routinely testing recipients for alloantibodies, unless there is academic interest in the possible pathogenic mechanism in individual TRALI cases.[34,36] Moreover, the widespread routine use of leukocyte reduction will probably reduce the likelihood of this type of reaction.

   e. The decision to further investigate and test donors associated with equivocal or non-life-threatening cases of

TRALI or possible TRALI should be determined after consultation between the blood center and the transfusion service physician. Although it may seem inconsistent to decide whether to investigate donors on the basis of the clinical severity of a case, it is frequently very difficult to recognize mild to moderate clinical manifestations that may represent TRALI.[5] As is the case with possible TRALI, the value of extensive investigation and donor deferral is unclear when the primary diagnosis of TRALI is not definitive. If these cases are investigated, all donors should usually be evaluated. However, an argument could be made for selectively testing donors for alloreactive leukocyte antibodies on the basis of the number and characteristics (eg, gender and parity) of the donors and components involved (see Recommendation 4 next). Similarly, Fadeyi et al[26] urge the investigation of transfusion reactions that do not fulfill the diagnostic criteria of TRALI if there is evidence of concomitant neutropenia with the transfusion.

4. **Evaluate donors.** Once a decision is made to investigate transfusion reactions associated with ALI, the evaluation should include all the components transfused within 6 hours before the onset of the reaction, and the following information should be documented:

    a. The blood components (eg, high vs low plasma-volume components) and their temporal association with the symptoms.

    b. The number of associated donors.

    c. The gender, pregnancy, and/or transfusion history of the associated donors.

    d. The duration of time between the transfusion of each blood component and the onset of symptoms (eg, transfusion within 2 hours of onset).

    e. Records of transfusion reactions linked to prior donations by the associated donors.

Investigation for alloreactive leukocyte antibodies may be performed on retention samples stored at the time of donation, on segments from the components involved in the reaction, or, preferably (and more commonly), on fresh samples collected from the donor during the investigation. If samples are derived from the residual transfused component returned to the blood center from the transfusion service, care should be taken in the interpretation of data because samples may have been contaminated or diluted after the reaction. Laboratory investigation for alloreactive leukocyte antibodies should include a screening test for both HLA Class I and II antibodies, as well as a test for HNA antibodies. Although some blood centers have used a staged approach of first determining the presence of HLA antibodies and then only testing components that are negative for HNA antibodies, this approach is not recommended by a number of experts in the field.[1,13,37] Positive screening test results should be complemented with an assay to determine the specificity of each antibody, a direct crossmatch test with recipient leukocytes, or both. If no recipient crossmatch is feasible, every effort should be made to determine the recipient HLA and HNA type, so that a determination of cognate recognition can be accomplished.[35]

5. **Plan for donor management.** Blood centers should have consistent criteria for managing donors associated with TRALI. The following actions have been recommended by experts in the field and have been variably implemented in US blood centers:

   a. Donors implicated in a case of TRALI should be permanently deferred from the donation of all transfusable blood components[1,4] (currently implemented in 95% of US blood centers and 44% of hospital blood banks).[13] Some authors have suggested that these donors may still safely donate red cells that are washed or that are frozen and deglycerolized before use; however, this proviso for individual exceptions is not practical in a large blood center.[1]

   b. Donors with specific HNA antibodies should be indefinitely deferred from all blood donation, regardless of their association with, or implication in, a TRALI case. Evidence suggests that specific HNA antibodies, especially HNA-3a antibodies, are most closely associated with severe TRALI and with milder reactions that are often not reported.[5,18,34,35]

c. Donors who harbor HLA or nonspecific HNA antibodies that are associated with a case of TRALI, but who are excluded from causation by crossmatch or recipient typing studies, may be redirected to donating low plasma-volume components. The role of nonspecific HNA antibodies in TRALI is particularly unclear, and some authors have suggested that these donors may continue to donate all components, especially if the antibodies have weak reactivity.[34] This alternate approach appears to be reasonable as long as the donors are tracked in such a manner that any future association with a second case of TRALI will lead to deferral.

d. If associated with TRALI by demonstration of HLA and/ or HNA antibodies, but not implicated because of the lack of a recipient type or crossmatch, donors should be deferred indefinitely from future donation (currently implemented in 78% of US blood centers and 8% of hospital blood banks).[4]

e. If associated with, but not implicated in, a case of TRALI resulting from an inability to test the donor for alloantibodies, the donor should be deferred from donation until such testing can be performed.

f. Donors associated with TRALI cases should be flagged in the computer system, and every investigation should include a review of the blood center records for association with prior transfusion reactions. The FDA BPAC has recommended that donors associated with two TRALI cases should be indefinitely deferred.[4]

g. If only one donor is associated with a TRALI case, consideration should be given to indefinite deferral regardless of whether an alloreactive antibody is detected, depending on the strength of the TRALI diagnosis, whether the product was a high plasma-volume component, and the amount of time between the transfusion and the reaction (currently implemented in 34% of US blood centers and 6% of hospital blood banks).[4,34]

h. Donors associated with a case of TRALI who are found to be negative for HLA and HNA antibodies should be allowed to continue to donate blood and components.

Conclusion

Investigations into the prevalence of HLA and HNA alloantibodies, the development of animal models of TRALI, and prospective studies on the incidence and risk factors for TRALI in clinical practice[19,38-41] are rapidly providing new insights into the mechanism of TRALI and may suggest possible interventions to decrease the risk to patients. A major limitation remains the lack of rapid, sensitive, specific, and inexpensive tests for HLA and HNA antibodies and the lack of sound scientific data linking specific antibodies to clinical TRALI. Increased focus in this area is stimulating the development of such tests and investigations. These endeavors will help the transfusion medicine community to prescribe a standard approach to the management of donors associated with, or implicated in, TRALI reactions that is based on scientific data. In the past, blood center physicians have made value judgments on the appropriate management of donors associated with TRALI by balancing the loss of donors against the perceived risk of continued donation. There is an urgent need—highlighted by the recognition of increased reporting of TRALI—to develop standardized and consistent approaches to donor investigation and management, with deferral criteria mandated through consensus standard-setting by the transfusion medicine community. The recommendations in this chapter may provide the framework for further deliberations.

References

1. Kleinman S, Caulfield T, Chan P, et al. Toward an understanding of transfusion-related acute lung injury: Statement of a consensus panel. Transfusion 2004; 44:1774-89.

2. Toy P, Popovsky MA, Abraham E, et al. Transfusion-related acute lung injury: Definition and review. Crit Care Med 2005;33:721-6.
3. Andrzejewski C, Popovsky MA. Transfusion-associated adverse pulmonary sequelae: Widening our perspective. Transfusion 2005;45:1048-50.
4. Englefreit CP, Reesink HW, Wendel S, et al. Measures to prevent TRALI. Vox Sang 2007;92:258-77.
5. Kopko PM, Marshall CS, MacKenzie MR, et al. Transfusion-related acute lung injury: Report of a clinical look-back investigation. JAMA 2002;287:1968-71.
6. Cooling L. Transfusion-related acute lung injury. JAMA 2002;288:315-16.
7. Dry SM, Bechard KM, Milford EL, et al. The pathology of transfusion-related acute lung injury. Am J Clin Pathol 1999;112:216-21.
8. Silliman CC, Ambruso DR, Boshkov LK. Transfusion-related acute lung injury. Blood 2005;105:2266-73.
9. Price TH, ed. Standards for blood banks and transfusion services. 25th ed. Bethesda, MD: AABB, 2008.
10. Final interim standard for *Standards for Blood Banks and Transfusion Services*, 23rd ed. Association bulletin #05-06. Bethesda, MD: AABB, 2005. [Available at http://www.aabb.org/Content/Members_Area/Association_Bulletins/ab05-6.htm (accessed June 28, 2008).]
11. Transfusion-related acute lung injury. Association bulletin #06-07. Bethesda, MD:AABB, 2006 [Available at http://www.aabb.org/Content/Members_Area/Association_Bulletins/ab06-07.htm (accessed June 28, 2008).]
12. Eder AF, Herron R, Strupp A, et al. Transfusion-related acute lung injury surveillance (2003-2005) and the potential impact of the selective use of plasma from male donors in the American Red Cross. Transfusion 2007;47:599-607.
13. Kopko P, Silva M, Shulman I, Kleinman S. AABB survey of transfusion-related acute lung injury policies and practices in the United States. Transfusion 2007;47:1679-85.
14. Silliman CC. The two-event model of transfusion-related acute lung injury. Crit Care Med 2006;34(5 Suppl):S124-31.
15. Popovsky MA. Transfusion and the lung: Circulatory overload and acute lung injury. Vox Sang 2004;87(Suppl 2):62-5.
16. Popovsky MA, Haley NR. Further characterization of transfusion-related acute lung injury: Demographics, clinical and laboratory features, and morbidity. Immunohematology 2001;17:157-9.
17. Popovsky MA, Moore SB. Diagnostic and pathogenetic considerations in transfusion-related acute lung injury. Transfusion 1985;25:573-7.
18. Davoren A, Curtis BR, Shulman IA, et al. TRALI due to granulocyte-agglutinating human neutrophil antigen-3a (5b) alloantibodies in donor plasma: A report of 2 fatalities. Transfusion 2003;43:641-5.
19. Triulzi DJ, Kakaiya R, Schreiber G. Donor risk factors for white blood cell antibodies associated with transfusion-associated acute lung injury: REDS-II leukocyte antibody prevalence study (LAPS). Transfusion 2007;47:563-4.
20. Triulzi D, Kakaiya R, Kleinman S, et al. Relationship of HLA antibodies in blood donors to pregnancy and transfusion history. Transfusion 2007;47 (Suppl 3):P4-030A.
21. Kao GS, Wood IG, Dorfman DM, et al. Investigations into the role of anti-HLA Class II antibodies in TRALI. Transfusion 2003;43:185-91.

22. Densmore TL, Goodnough LT, Ali S, et al. Prevalence of HLA sensitization in female apheresis donors. Transfusion 1999;39:103-6.

23. Kleinman S. A perspective on transfusion-related acute lung injury two years after the Canadian Consensus Conference. Transfusion 2006;46:1465-8.

24. Nicolle AL, Chapman CE, Carter V, Wallis JP. Transfusion-related acute lung injury caused by two donors with anti-human leucocyte antigen Class II antibodies: A look-back investigation. Transfus Med 2004;14:225-30.

25. Win N, Ranasinghe E, Lucas G. Transfusion-related acute lung injury: A 5-year look-back study. Transfus Med 2002;12:387-9.

26. Fadeyi EA, De Los Angeles Muniz M, Wayne AS, et al. The transfusion of neutrophil-specific antibodies causes leukopenia and a broad spectrum of pulmonary reactions. Transfusion 2007;47:545-50.

27. Toy P, Hollis-Perry KM, Jun J, Nakagawa M. Recipients of blood from a donor with multiple HLA antibodies: A lookback study of transfusion-related acute lung injury. Transfusion 2004;44:1683-8.

28. Zupanska B, Uhrynowska M, Michur H, et al. Transfusion-related acute lung injury and leucocyte-reacting antibodies. Vox Sang 2007;93:70-7.

29. Triulzi DJ. Transfusion-related acute lung injury: An update. Hematology Am Soc Hematol Educ Program 2006:497-501.

30. O'Riordan T, Cameron J. Interpreting the precautionary principle. London: Earthscan Publications Ltd, 1994.

31. Webert KE, Blajchman MA. Transfusion-related acute lung injury. Transfus Med Rev 2003;17:252-62.

32. Popovsky MA, Chaplin HC Jr, Moore SB. Transfusion-related acute lung injury: A neglected, serious complication of hemotherapy. Transfusion 1992;32:589-92.

33. Kopko PM, Popovsky MA, MacKenzie MR, et al. HLA Class II antibodies in transfusion-related acute lung injury. Transfusion 2001;41:1244-8.

34. Su L, Kamel H. How do we investigate and manage donors associated with a suspected case of transfusion-related acute lung injury? Transfusion 2007;47:1118-24.

35. Stroncek DF, Fadeyi E, Adams S. Leukocyte antigen and antibody detection assays: Tools for assessing and preventing pulmonary transfusion reactions. Transfus Med Rev 2007;21:273-86.

36. Kleinman S, Gajic O, Nunes E. Promoting recognition and prevention of transfusion-related acute lung injury. Crit Care Nurse 2007;27:49-53.

37. Bux J. Transfusion-related acute lung injury (TRALI): A serious adverse event of blood transfusion. Vox Sang 2005;89:1-10.

38. Looney MR, Su X, Van Ziffle JA, et al. Neutrophils and their Fc gamma receptors are essential in a mouse model of transfusion-related acute lung injury. J Clin Invest 2006;116:1615-23.

39. Looney MR, Matthay MA. Animal models of transfusion-related acute lung injury. Crit Care Med 2006;34(5 Suppl):S132-6.

40. Rana R, Fernandez-Perez ER, Khan SA, et al. Transfusion-related acute lung injury and pulmonary edema in critically ill patients: A retrospective study. Transfusion 2006;46:1478-83.

41. Gajic O, Rana R, Mendez JL, et al. Acute lung injury after blood transfusion in mechanically ventilated patients. Transfusion 2004;44:1468-74.

In: Kleinman S, Popovsky MA, eds.
TRALI: Mechanisms, Management, and Prevention
Bethesda, MD: AABB Press, 2008

5

HLA Antibody Testing

PATRICIA M. KOPKO, MD

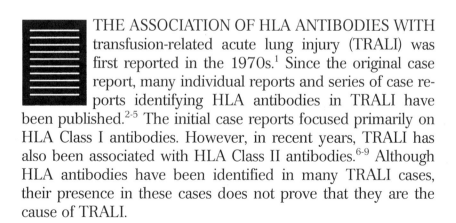 THE ASSOCIATION OF HLA ANTIBODIES WITH transfusion-related acute lung injury (TRALI) was first reported in the 1970s.[1] Since the original case report, many individual reports and series of case reports identifying HLA antibodies in TRALI have been published.[2-5] The initial case reports focused primarily on HLA Class I antibodies. However, in recent years, TRALI has also been associated with HLA Class II antibodies.[6-9] Although HLA antibodies have been identified in many TRALI cases, their presence in these cases does not prove that they are the cause of TRALI.

Patricia M. Kopko, MD, Executive Vice President, Medical Affairs, and Director, Histocompatibility Laboratory, BloodSource, Mather, California

HLA Antibodies and TRALI

When both members of the donor/recipient pair are tested for HLA antibodies, HLA antibodies are identified in approximately 70% of TRALI cases.[2] In 85% to 90% of the cases, the antibody is identified in the blood component transfused. In approximately 10% of cases, the antibody is identified in the transfusion recipient.[1-3] In rare case reports, antibody in a transfused blood component corresponds to an HLA antigen present in another blood component transfused to the same recipient.[10-12] Such infrequent cases of TRALI have been termed "interdonor TRALI."

HLA antibodies can be formed after exposure to foreign HLA proteins. The three potential routes of exposure to HLA alloantigens are pregnancy, transfusion, and transplantation. The most common source of HLA antibodies in healthy blood donors is pregnancy. A recent study of blood components demonstrated the presence of HLA Class I or HLA Class II antibodies, or both, in 22% of the components tested.[13] If approximately one-fifth of blood components contain HLA antibodies, and if the presence of antibody alone were sufficient to cause TRALI, the disorder would be much more common than currently observed. There is a growing appreciation that antibodies alone are not sufficient to cause TRALI and that the etiology of TRALI is complex. There is also a growing appreciation that HLA antibodies represent an important factor in the pathogenesis of TRALI (see Chapter 3).

To prove that HLA antibodies can cause TRALI in some patients, a controlled outcome study of patients who receive blood components with HLA antibodies that correspond to their HLA proteins would need to be performed. Yet such a study would be impossible to execute because of ethical concerns, given that the infusion of HLA-DR antibody in an experimental study designed to mimic hemolytic disease of the fetus and newborn resulted in a clinical case of TRALI in the study subject.[7] Data from other types of studies are available, however. Based on the association of HLA antibodies with TRALI and a clear association of TRALI with plasma from female donors, the United Kingdom National Blood Service implemented a strategy in late 2003 to attempt to reduce the incidence of TRALI.[14,15] Throughout the United Kingdom, plasma for transfusion was manufactured predominantly from male donors. In addition, platelet concentrates were resuspended predominantly in plasma from male donors. No changes were made in the gender of apheresis platelet donors; however, 70% of the apheresis platelet donors were male.

Although the efforts to switch to all-male plasma commenced at the end of 2003, female plasma was still available for transfusion in 2004 because female plasma was still in transfusion services inventories at the beginning of the year, and the transition to predominantly male plasma became effective over time. In 2006, 86% of platelet pools and plasma were produced from male donors.[14] Since the implementation of this risk reduction strategy, both the number of reports of TRALI and the number of deaths at least possibly caused by TRALI have decreased by 73% and 86%, respectively. Additionally, TRALI cases secondary to the transfusion of plasma with proven relevant antibody (antibody in the donor against cognate antigen in the recipient) have decreased from 10 cases in 2003 to none in 2005 or 2006. TRALI cases secondary to the transfusion of platelets involving a relevant antibody have decreased from 8 cases in 2003 to 3 cases in 2005 and 1 case in 2006 (see Chapter 7).

The American Red Cross performed a retrospective study of TRALI case reports from 2003 to 2005 in order to evaluate the association of white blood cell antibodies and gender with fatalities.[16] A total of 550 suspected cases of TRALI were reported. Of these cases, 72 involved fatalities. Reports were analyzed to classify cases as "probable TRALI" or as "unrelated etiology." Of the 72 fatalities, 38 were classified as probable TRALI. Transfusion of plasma was involved in 24 of the 38 (63%) cases, with an additional 5 cases (13%) occurring after the transfusion of apheresis platelets. A female with white blood cell antibodies was identified in 27 of 38 (71%) fatal cases and in 18 of 24 (75%) cases occurring after plasma transfusion. Antibody-positive female donors were significantly more likely to be associated with probable TRALI cases than with unrelated etiology cases (p <0.0001). Compared to red cell components, plasma was 12.5 times more likely to be associated with probable TRALI, whereas apheresis platelets were 7.9 times more likely to be associated with probable TRALI.

In response to these and other studies, the AABB released *Association Bulletins* #06-07 and #07-03.[17,18] These bulletins recommend a two-pronged approach to reduce the risk of TRALI. The first recommendation is to minimize the transfusion of high plasma-volume components (plasma and apheresis platelets) from leukocyte-alloimmunized donors. The second recommendation is to minimize the inappropriate transfusion of blood components. Member facilities are encouraged to choose specific strategies in order to work toward achieving these objectives while balancing the risk of TRALI with the need to maintain an adequate blood supply. Strategies to minimize the transfusion of plasma from leukocyte-alloimmunized donors were recommended to be in place by November 2007.

Because the volume of plasma needed for transfusion is significantly less than the amount collected every year, many blood centers in the United States have implemented the recommendation in the AABB *Bulletins* by providing male-only or predominantly male plasma. Instead of using plasma from female donors for transfusion, female plasma is used to manufacture albumin, intravenous immune globulin, and other important medications. Because of the excess of plasma for transfusion in the United States, the implementation of male-only or predominantly male plasma programs has been relatively easy and has been approached from the perspective of inventory management. Strategies to minimize the transfusion of platelets from alloimmunized donors are recommended to begin by November 2008. Because there is no excess in the supply of platelets, the implementation of male-only or predominantly male platelet programs will be more difficult and will have the potential to jeopardize the supply of platelets. Therefore, many centers are considering testing either donors with a history of pregnancy or all female donors for the presence of HLA antibodies.

The HLA System

The genes of the HLA system are located within the major histocompatibility complex (MHC) on the short arm of chromosome 6. The MHC comprises more than 200 genes. For the purposes of TRALI, the most significant genes of the MHC are those that encode the HLA Class I and HLA Class II proteins. The primary functions of these proteins are antigen processing and presentation as well as recognition of self from nonself.[19]

HLA Class I proteins are present on most nucleated cells and platelets (the product of nucleated megakaryocytes). These proteins are not typically present on mature red cells. The HLA Class I region of the MHC is comprised of the classical genes *HLA-A, HLA-B,* and *HLA-C* and the nonclassical genes *HLA-E, HLA-F, HLA-G, HFE, HLA-J, HLA-K, HLA-L, MICA,* and *MICAB.*[20] Antibodies to the HLA-A and HLA-B antigens have been associated with TRALI.[21] Antibodies to all other MHC Class I proteins (both classical and nonclassical) have not been associated with TRALI.

HLA Class I molecules are composed of a transmembrane glycoprotein α heavy chain and β_2 microglobulin. β_2 microglobulin is not encoded in the MHC. The β_2 microglobulin gene is present on chromosome 15. The α polypeptide chain comprises five domains (Fig 5-1).[19] Three of the five domains are extracellular. Those are the $\alpha1$ and $\alpha2$ peptide binding domains and the $\alpha3$ immunoglobulin-like domain. The remaining two domains of the α polypeptide are the transmembrane and intracellular domains.

HLA Class II proteins are expressed on fewer cell types than are HLA Class I proteins. The HLA Class II proteins are found primarily on a variety of immune cells, including B cells, activated T cells, dendritic cells, and macrophages. Other cell types can be induced to express HLA Class II molecules by interferon-8.[19] The HLA Class II region of the MHC encodes for HLA-DR, HLA-DQ, and HLA-DP proteins. HLA-DR and HLA-DQ have been associated with TRALI.[21]

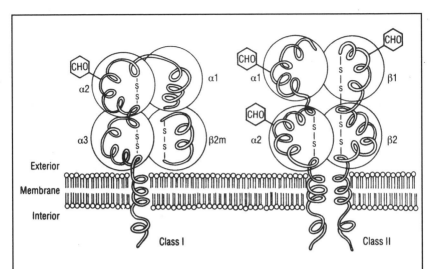

Figure 5-1. Stylized diagram of Class I and Class II MHC molecules show-ing α and β polypeptide chains, their structural domains, and attached car-bohydrate units. (Reprinted with permission from Gebel et al.[20])

HLA Class II molecules comprise two similar (α and β) glyco-protein chains. The α and β glycoprotein chains each comprise four domains (Fig 5-1). Each has two extracellular domains (peptide binding and immunoglobulin-like), a transmembrane domain, and an intracellular domain. The outermost or peptide binding domain contains the variable regions of the HLA Class II molecules.

Historically, HLA antibodies have been divided into antisera to private epitopes and antisera to public epitopes. Functionally, antisera to private epitopes identified a single HLA molecule (eg, HLA-A1). Antisera that reacted with multiple HLA antigens (eg, HLA-A1, -A3, -A11, and -A36) identified public epitopes.[22]

The term "public epitope" is often used interchangeably with "cross-reactive group (CREG)." Technically, this interpretation is incorrect. All of the HLA Class I specificities can be divided into CREGs (Table 5-1). However, more than one public epitope can be present in a single CREG. This concept explains why an indi-vidual with a single allogeneic exposure can make antibodies to a single antigen, to a subset of antigens from a CREG, or to an

Table 5-1. Cross-Reactive Groups

Group	HLA Class I Specificities
1C	A1, A3, A11, A29, A30, A31, A36, A80
2C	A2, A23, A24, A68, A69, B57, B58
4C	A23, A24, A25, A32, B_w4
5C	B18, B35, B46, B49, B50, B51, B52, B53, B62, B63, B71, B72, B73, B75, B76, B77, B78
6C	B_w6
7C	B7, B8, B13, B27, B41, B42, B47, B48, B54, B55, B56, B59, B60, B61, B67, B81, B82
8C	B8, B18, B38, B39, B59, B64, B65, B67
10C	A25, A26, A32, A33, A34, A43, A66, A74
12C	B13, B37, B41, B44, B45, B47, B49, B50, B60, B61

entire CREG.[22] Additionally, because a single allogeneic exposure can present multiple foreign HLA antigens (eg, 2 HLA-A, 2 HLA-B, 2 HLA-C, 2 HLA-DR, and 2 HLA-DQ), a large number of antibodies can be formed after a single pregnancy, transplantation, or transfusion.

The nomenclature of the HLA system can resemble a random group of letters and numbers. The letter(s) correspond(s) to the HLA locus. The first 2 digits after the letter correspond to the HLA antigen within the locus. The antigens were numbered in the order they were discovered. Thus, in general, HLA antigens with a low number tend to occur more frequently than do HLA antigens with a higher number. When an HLA assignment is reported as a letter followed by one or two numbers (eg, *HLA-A23*), this represents an antigen level typing. This level of typing was the most common typing available until the widespread availability of molecular typing. With molecular typing, it quickly became apparent that there were many different alleles of each of the HLA antigens. In HLA nomenclature, an asterisk is placed after the letter(s) to represent a molecular type. Like the antigenic designations, the HLA alleles were assigned numbers in the order in which they were identified. Thus, *HLA-A*2304* is the fourth allele of *HLA-A23* identified. Also similar to the antigenic nomenclature, alleles with low numbers tend to be more common than alleles with high numbers.

HLA Class II nomenclature is very similar to Class I nomenclature. In addition to the combination of letters and numbers used for Class I, the symbols α and β are used to designate the two polypeptide chains. Thus, *HLA-DRβ 0103* designates the β chain of the *HLA-DR 0103* allele.

Methodologies for HLA Antibody Detection

Overview

At first glance, testing for HLA antibodies can appear very complex. However, once it is appreciated that all of the test methodologies are exceedingly similar, a basic understanding of the testing is achieved. Such a foundation allows for a more thorough understanding of the different test methodologies as well as for a comprehension of the pros and cons of using each technique for blood-donor screening.

Test kits for the detection of HLA antibodies are commercially available for several testing methodologies. Methodologies include complement-dependent cytotoxicity (CDC), the enzyme-linked immunosorbent assay (ELISA), flow cytometry, and Luminex (Luminex Corp, Austin, TX). Each of these tests consists of a first incubation, followed by a wash, and then a second incubation, followed by a wash. The final assay step is a detection phase. (See Fig 5-2.)

In the initial incubation phase, donor serum or plasma is incubated with target HLA antigens. Depending on the methodology used, the target HLA antigens are present on cells, the test well, or microparticles (see Table 5-2). This incubation allows any antibody that is directed against a target HLA antigen to

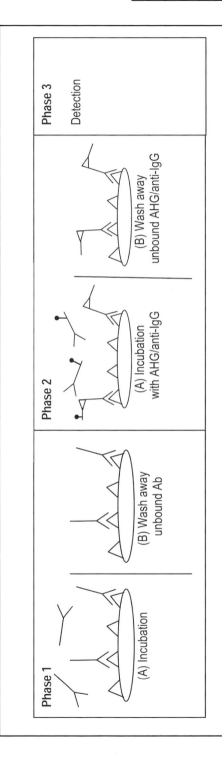

Figure 5-2. Phases of HLA antibody detection methodologies. Phase 1: Serum is incubated with HLA antigens bound on cells, test wells, or microparticle beads (A), and unbound antibody is washed away (B). Phase 2: Antihuman globulin (AHG) or anti-IgG is incubated with the test system (A), and unbound antibody is washed away (B). Phase 3: The presence of AHG or anti-IgG is detected according to different methodologies (see Table 5-2).

Table 5-2. HLA Antibody Screening Methodologies

Method	Surface	Anti-IgG Labeled with	Detection	Instrumentation
CDC	Cells	N/A (complement enhances AHG)	Cell death	Microscope
ELISA	Antigen-coated wells	Enzyme	Color change	Luminometer
Flow cytometry	Antigen-coated beads	Fluorescent label	Fluorescence	Flow cytometer
Luminex	Antigen-coated beads	Fluorescent label	Fluorescence	Luminex

CDC = complement-dependent cytotoxicity; N/A = not applicable; AHG = antihuman globulin; ELISA = enzyme-linked immunosorbent assay.

bind. After the first incubation phase, a wash step is used to remove any unbound antibody.

Antihuman globulin (AHG) or anti-IgG is added to the test system before a second incubation. During the second incubation, AHG or anti-IgG binds to any donor antibody that is bound to the target HLA antigens. At least one more wash step is used to remove any unbound antibody.

The final phase of these tests involves the detection of bound AHG or anti-IgG. Each of the tests uses different instrumentation to detect the presence of AHG or anti-IgG. In the cytotoxic method, complement is added, and the presence of AHG is detected by microscopic visualization of cell death. In the ELISA, an enzyme is conjugated to the anti-IgG, and a substrate is added to the test system. The enzyme acts on the substrate, resulting in a detectable change to the test. The change is often in the color of the test well, which can easily be detected by a spectrophotometer. In flow cytometry and Luminex, the anti-IgG is labeled with a fluorescent tag. In both methodologies, a laser is used to excite the fluorescent tag, which releases energy in the form of photons. The photons are detected by a photomultiplier tube.

Complement-Dependent Cytotoxicity

CDC is a cellular-based assay that relies on cell death to detect the presence of antibodies. Complement is used in the test system to cause cell death through activation of the complement cascade. CDC is the least sensitive of the methodologies used to detect HLA antibodies.

Many modifications of the test steps can be made depending on the sensitivity desired[23]; such modifications include the number of washes, length of incubation, and addition of AHG. In general, each of these modifications will make the test more sensitive.

Although the reagents or test kits used for CDC can be inexpensive, the testing is entirely manual and requires significant technical expertise to perform and interpret. Commercial test kits are available, but they have largely fallen out of use in the United States because of their complexity.

Test trays typically have 30 to 50 wells. Each well contains cells—and thus HLA antigens—derived from a single individual. An entire tray must be used to screen a single sample. When the trays are made, careful consideration must be given to ensure that all of the antigens that need to be detected are adequately represented. Because there is substantial variation between HLA antigens in various ethnic groups, consideration also needs to be given to ensuring that the antigens on the test tray represent the ethnicity of antibodies likely present in the population being screened.

CDC can be used both for HLA antibody screening and for identification of antibody specificity, if the panel size is large enough. T-cells or unfractionated lymphocytes can be used to detect HLA Class I antibodies. Because HLA Class II molecules are not present on unactivated T-cells, B-cells are required to screen for HLA Class II antibodies.

One of the biggest obstacles to using CDC for blood donor screening is that the test is not specific for HLA antibodies. Other antibodies directed against proteins present on the surface of lymphocytes can result in a positive test result if corresponding antigens are present.

The CDC test has been widely used in histocompatibility laboratories to screen potential solid organ transplant recipients for HLA antibodies. In recent years, the CDC test has been used less frequently and is being replaced by noncellular methods. The CDC test does not adapt well to blood donor screening because of the labor-intensive nature of CDC testing and its interpretation.

ELISA

ELISA testing for HLA antibodies is very similar to the ELISA used by blood centers for viral marker testing for blood. Commercial test kits are readily available. Testing trays contain multiple wells. HLA antigens are isolated and bound to the test wells. The solid surface used in commercial test kits is antigen-coated wells.[24] The wells are coated with a full complement of HLA-A, HLA-B, HLA-DR, and HLA-DQ antigens. Positive and negative test results are determined by calculation of a sample/cutoff (S/CO) ratio. In general, two test wells are required to test a single sample: one for HLA Class I and one for HLA Class II. The test kits available require manual pipetting and wash steps. Manufacturers are working on automated testing equipment similar to equipment currently available in donor testing laboratories. ELISA is more sensitive than CDC but less sensitive than flow cytometry or Luminex. Because ELISA is a noncellular test, it does not detect non-HLA antibodies.

ELISA is very easy to interpret. Test results are either positive or negative according to a cutoff value. ELISA does not provide indeterminate test results. The familiarity of ELISA and its ease of interpretation make this test easily adaptable to blood donor screening.

Flow Cytometry

In the past decade, flow cytometry has become widely available to screen for HLA antibodies. Commercial test kits are available from multiple vendors.[25] The solid surface in this test is latex microparticle beads. The beads are coated with a variety of HLA Class I or II antigens. A number of antigen-coated beads are mixed to provide a full complement of HLA-A, HLA-B, HLA-DR, and HLA-DQ antigens in the test. The Class I and Class II beads can be distinguished in the flow cytometer because of different fluorescent labels. Thus, an antibody screen for both Class I and Class II can be performed in a single assay.

The test results are presented as histograms (see Fig 5-3). A negative result is typically a single well-defined peak that is similar or identical to the negative control. A positive result is typically a single peak or multiple peaks that are clearly shifted to a higher median channel (increased fluorescence) than the negative control and the negative beads in the sample. Flow cytome-

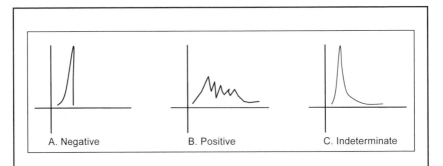

Figure 5-3. Representation of test results for flow cytometry HLA antibody screening: Negative, single well-defined peak (A). Positive, multiple peaks shifted to higher median channel (B). Indeterminate, single peak with "shoulder" on right side (higher median channel) of peak (C).

try can result in indeterminate test results. An indeterminate test result is one that is neither clearly negative nor clearly positive. In most indeterminate results, a single peak with a "shoulder" is shifted to a higher median channel. If indeterminate test results on a screening test are followed up with more specific testing, the results can subsequently be classified as either positive or negative. Flow cytometry is very sensitive and can detect HLA antibodies that are too weak to be demonstrated by cytotoxic crossmatch. Because flow cytometry is a noncellular test, it is specific for HLA antibodies.

Interpretation of test results is typically based on visual analysis. The test setup involves several manual steps, among them pipetting and washing. Although data acquisition is performed by the flow cytometer, many manual computer steps must be performed during this analysis. Maintenance for a flow cytometer, data acquisition, and data analysis are complex and require significant experience and expertise. Although flow cytometry is used successfully in many histocompatibility laboratories, the manual nature of the test methodology and data interpretation are not highly compatible with the high-volume testing required for blood component processing.

Luminex

Luminex is very similar to flow cytometry. The principles involved in the functioning of the instrumentation are identical to those of flow cytometry.[26] The primary differences are that Luminex is a much smaller instrument, is easier to operate, and is easier to maintain than a flow cytometer. Therefore, the level of technical expertise needed is less than that required for flow cytometry.

Commercial test kits are available from multiple vendors. Like flow cytometry, the solid surface used in Luminex is microparticle beads. The beads are coated with HLA antigens. A full complement of HLA-A, HLA-B, HLA-Cw, HLA-DR, and HLA-DQ antigens is present in the screening test. Like flow cytometry, differences in fluorescent labeling between the HLA Class I and HLA Class II beads allow the instrumentation to distinguish between the beads. Thus, screening for HLA Class I and HLA Class II antibodies can be performed in a single test. The test results are presented in a numeric fashion. The cutoff between positive and negative can be set by using a predetermined value or can be determined individually by each laboratory. Because a numeric cutoff is used, there are no indeterminate test results. Luminex is extremely sensitive. Because it is a noncellular test, Luminex is specific for HLA antibodies.

Currently, the test system is labor-intensive, with manual pipetting and washing steps. Test manufacturers are in the process of developing automated equipment to greatly reduce the amount of labor required to perform this test. The ease of testing, interpretation, and equipment operation may make this test well suited to blood donor screening.

Conclusion

The limited supply of platelets available for transfusion makes conversion to a predominantly male or an all-male base of platelet apheresis donors impractical for most blood collection facilities. Therefore, many organizations will implement HLA antibody screening of high-risk donors to reduce the risk of TRALI from apheresis platelets.

A number of commercially available test systems are capable of detecting HLA antibodies. Methodologies available include CDC, ELISA, flow cytometry, and Luminex. These tests have been used in histocompatibility laboratories, primarily for screening potential organ recipients for HLA antibodies. Traditionally, identification of HLA antibodies against a specific HLA antigen would prohibit transplantation of a solid organ to a recipient with the cognate antigen. However, improved immunosuppressive protocols, combined with the ability to detect very low levels of HLA antibodies with newer testing methodologies, have expanded the consideration of what is considered an "acceptable mismatch."[27]

The challenges for blood collection facilities in implementing HLA antibody screening will be numerous. First, this testing was designed to support solid organ transplantation, not apheresis donor screening. Therefore, testing facilities will need to consider how to adapt this testing to the higher throughput that may be required for the screening of platelet apheresis donors. Second, the available assays do not have current good manufacturing practice (cGMP) controls, which are standard in other blood-donor screening assay systems. Facilities will need to implement manual control points to ensure compliance with cGMPs. This implementation may include determination of the assay cutoff (ie, although most blood-donor screening tests perform an automatic calculation of the assay cutoff, some HLA antibody assays allow or require individual laboratory determination of the appropriate cutoff). Third, HLA antibody screening tests are relatively new and have been used primarily in the specific clinical setting of organ transplantation. Furthermore, the tests have been applied in a nonstandardized fashion by transplantation laboratories and transplantation centers so that general understanding of their utility and optimization in organ transplantation is still evolving. Blood collection facilities need to keep this in mind when extrapolating results from the organ transplantation (ie, diagnostic) setting to the very different setting of determining donor eligibility for platelet apheresis. It is thus likely that modifications will need to be made to some of these assay systems as they are applied to testing apheresis donors; the required modifications may be determined only after additional experience has been gained in this screening setting.

References

1. Wolf CFW, Canale VC. Fatal pulmonary hypersensitivity reaction to HLA-A incompatible blood transfusion: Report of a case and review of the literature. Transfusion 1976;16:135-40.

2. Popovsky MA, Moore SB. Diagnostic and pathogenetic considerations in transfusion-related acute lung injury. Transfusion 1985;25:573-7.

3. Kopko PM, Paglierioni TG, Popovsky MA, et al. TRALI: Correlation of antigen-antibody and monocytes activation in donor-recipient pairs. Transfusion 2003; 43:177-84.

4. Dykes A, Smallwood D, Kotsimbos T, Street A. Transfusion-related acute lung injury (TRALI) in a patient with a single lung transplant. Br J Haematol 2000;109:671-8.

5. Popovsky MA, Haley NR. Further characterization of transfusion-related acute lung injury: Demographics, clinical and laboratory features, and morbidity. Immunohematology 2000;16:157-9.

6. Kopko PM, Popovsky MA, MacKenzie MR, et al. Human leukocyte antigen class II antibodies in transfusion-related acute lung injury. Transfusion 2001; 41:1244-8.

7. Flesch BK, Neppert J. Transfusion-related acute lung injury caused by human leucocyte antigen class II antibody. Br J Haematol 2002;116:673-6.

8. Kao GS, Wood IG, Dorfman DM, et al. Investigations into the role of anti-HLA class II antibodies in TRALI. Transfusion 2003;43:185-91.

9. Nicolle AL, Chapman CE, Carter V, Wallis P. Transfusion-related acute lung injury caused by two donors with anti-human leucocyte antigen class II antibodies: A look-back investigation. Transfus Med 2004;64:225-30.

10. Eastlund DT, McGrath PC, Burkart P. Platelet transfusion reaction associated with interdonor HLA incompatibility. Vox Sang 1988;55:157-60.

11. O'Connor JC, Strauss RG, Goeken NE, Knox LB. A near-fatal reaction during granulocyte transfusion of a neonate. Transfusion 1988;28:173-6.

12. Virchis AE, Patel RK, Contreras M, et al. Acute non-cardiogenic lung edema after platelet transfusion. Br Med J 1997;314:880-2.

13. Bray RA, Harris SB, Josephson CD, et al. Unappreciated risk factors for transplant patients: HLA antibodies in blood components. Hum Immunol 2004; 65:240-4.

14. Serious Hazards of Transfusion (SHOT) annual report 2006. Manchester, UK: SHOT Scheme, 2007. [Available at http://www.shotuk.org/SHOT_report_2006.pdf (accessed June 30, 2008).]

15. Wendel S, Biagini S, Trigo F, et al. Measures to prevent TRALI. Vox Sang 2007;92:258-77.

16. Eder AF, Herron R, Strupp A, et al. Transfusion-related acute lung injury surveillance (2003-2005) and the potential impact of the selective use of plasma from male donors in the American Red Cross. Transfusion 2007;47:599-607.

17. Transfusion-related acute lung injury. Association bulletin #06-07. Bethesda, MD: AABB, 2006. [Available at http://www.aabb.org/Content/Members_Area/Association_Bulletins/ab06-07.htm (accessed June 30, 2008).]

18. Clarifications to recommendations to reduce the risk of TRALI. Association bulletin #07-03. Bethesda, MD: AABB, 2007. [Available at http://www.aabb.org/Content/Members_Area/Association_Bulletins/ab07-03.htm (accessed June 30, 2008).]

19. Klein J, Sato A. The HLA system. N Engl J Med 2000;343:702-9.

20. Gebel HM, Pollack MS, Bray RA. The HLA system. In: Roback J, Combs MR, Grossman B, Hillyer C, eds. Technical manual. 16th ed. Bethesda, MD: AABB, 2008:547-68.

21. Kopko PM, Popovsky MA. Transfusion-related acute lung injury. In: Popovsky MA, ed. Transfusion reactions. 3rd ed. Bethesda, MD: AABB Press, 2007:207-28.

22. Rodey GE. HLA beyond tears: Introduction to human histocompatibility. 2nd ed. Durango, CO: De Novo, Inc, 2000.

23. Hopkins KA. The basic lymphocyte microcytotoxicity tests: Standard and AHG enhancement. In: Hahn AB, Land GA, Strothman R, eds. ASHI laboratory manual. 4th ed. Mt. Laurel, NJ: American Society of Histocompatibility and Immunogenetics, 2000.

24. Osowski LD, Gutierrez M, Muth B. HLA antibody screening and identification by ELISA methodology. In: Hahn AB, Land GA, Strothman R, eds. ASHI laboratory manual. 4th ed. Mt. Laurel, NJ: American Society of Histocompatibility and Immunogenetics, 2000.

25. Wilmoth-Hosey L, Bray RA. Antibody identification by flow cytometry using HLA class I or class II antigen coated specificity beads. In: Hahn AB, Land GA, Strothman R, eds. ASHI laboratory manual. 4th ed. Mt. Laurel, NJ: American Society of Histocompatibility and Immunogenetics, 2000.

26. Lefell MS, Bray RA. Basic principles and quality assurance of immunofluorescence and flow cytometry. In: Hahn AB, Land GA, Strothman R, eds. ASHI laboratory manual. 4th ed. Mt. Laurel, NJ: American Society of Histocompatibility and Immunogenetics, 2000.

27. Leffell MS, Montgomery RA, Zachary AA. The changing role of antibody testing in transplantation. Clin Transpl 2005:259-71.

In: Kleinman S, Popovsky MA, eds.
TRALI: Mechanisms, Management, and Prevention
Bethesda, MD: AABB Press, 2008

6

Detection of Neutrophil Antigens and Antibodies

DAVID F. STRONCEK, MD

LEUKOCYTE ANTIGENS WERE DESCRIBED more than 50 years ago using leukocyte agglutination assays. Classic leukoagglutinins included antibodies to HLA antigens and neutrophil-specific antigens. Neutrophil-specific antigens are known as human neutrophil antigens (HNA), which are made up of several unrelated molecules expressed predominantly, if not exclusively, by neutrophils. Antibodies to neutrophil antigens cause neonatal alloimmune neutropenia, autoimmune neutropenia of

David F. Stroncek, MD, Chief, Cell Processing Section, Department of Transfusion Medicine, Warren G. Magnuson Clinical Center, National Institutes of Health, Bethesda, Maryland childhood, and transfusion reactions, including transfusion-related acute lung injury (TRALI).

The identification of neutrophil antigens and of antibodies to these antigens is important for the evaluation of patients and donors involved in pulmonary transfusion reactions. In evaluating a transfusion reaction, it is important to determine if antibodies are present in the transfused blood component or blood donor. When neutrophil antibodies are detected, it is often necessary to determine if the antibody is specific to a neutrophil antigen and to identify the specific antigen to which the antibody is directed. It is also helpful to assess the neutrophil antigen type of the transfusion recipient in order to determine if the antibody is directed to an antigen expressed by the recipient. This chapter reviews neutrophil-specific antigens as well as methods to type these antigens and to detect antibodies to them. In addition, strategies to evaluate patients and donors implicated in transfusion reactions are discussed.

The Role of Neutrophil Antibodies in Transfusion Reactions

Antibodies to neutrophil and HLA antigens can cause a variety of transfusion reactions. These reactions include febrile transfusion reactions, pulmonary transfusion reactions in recipients of granulocyte concentrates, and pulmonary transfusion reactions in recipients of plasma-containing blood components.

Febrile Transfusion Reactions

In the 1950s, Brittingham found that the transfusion of whole blood into patients with leukoagglutinins could cause febrile reactions.[1] Both HLA and neutrophil-specific antibodies cause these reactions. Brittingham showed that these reactions could be prevented by removing the buffy coat from the whole blood.[1] The risks of such reactions can be reduced in frequency and severity by transfusing leukocyte-reduced Red Blood Cells (RBCs) and platelet components.[2-4]

Pulmonary Transfusion Reactions

Granulocyte transfusion recipients sometimes experience transfusion reactions characterized by shortness of breath, fever, and hemoglobin oxygen desaturation.[5-7] Chest x-rays in patients experiencing these reactions may reveal new or worsening pulmonary infiltrates, but the pulmonary dysfunction is usually mild to moderate in severity and resolves within a few hours. These reactions occur in granulocyte transfusion recipients alloimmunized to HLA Class I or neutrophil-specific antigens. Most often, they are caused by HLA antibodies.[5-7] These reactions are likely a result of antibody-antigen interactions that cause the transfused granulocytes to become trapped in the pulmonary capillaries, resulting in ventilation or perfusion mismatching and hypoxia.

Plasma-containing blood components can also cause pulmonary transfusion reactions. In 1957, Brittingham found that the transfusion of leukoagglutinins sometimes caused severe pulmonary transfusion reactions.[1] The transfusion of 50 mL of plasma with strong leukocyte agglutinins resulted in immediate faintness, followed in about 45 minutes by vomiting, diarrhea, chills, fever, severe hypotension, severe tachypnea, dyspnea, cyanosis, and initial leukopenia followed by leukocytosis. The next day, the transfusion recipient was comfortable, but a chest x-ray showed marked bilateral pulmonary infiltrates and a small pleural effusion. The x-ray abnormalities disappeared 3 days later.[1] Several cases of these "hypersensitivity" reactions were reported in the 1960s and 1970s.[8,9] In the 1980s, the term "transfusion-related acute lung injury," or TRALI, was first used by Popovsky and colleagues to describe these types of reactions, and the idea that antibodies to HLA Class I and neutrophil antigens were an important cause of TRALI became widely accepted.[10] Antibodies to HNA-1b,[11] HNA-2a,[12] and HNA-3a[13,14] have been implicated in TRALI.

Neutrophil Antigen Systems

Several clinically important neutrophil antigen systems are referred to as HNA systems.[15] The antigen systems are designated by integers, and specific antigens in each system are designated alphabetically by date of publication.[15] There are five HNA antigen systems: HNA-1, -2, -3, -4, and -5 (Table 6-1). These antigens are not as closely related as are the HLA antigens. In fact, HNA antigens are located on different molecules and are related only in their importance in neutrophil immunology.

HNA-1 Antigen System

The best characterized neutrophil antigen system is HNA-1, which has three alleles: *HNA-1a*, *HNA-1b*, and *HNA-1c*. The first allele was identified by Lalezari and Bernard in 1966 and was originally called *NA1*.[16] Boxer and colleagues identified another allele, *NA2*, in 1972.[17] These antigens are now known as HNA-1a and HNA-1b. HNA-1c was decribed by Bux et al in 1997.[18] The HNA-1 antigens are located on human neutrophil Fc-gamma-receptor IIIb (FcγRIIIb) (CD16) and encoded by the *FCGR3B* gene located on chromosome 1.[19] HNA-1 antigens are only located on neutrophils and, hence, are neutrophil-specific. However, soluble FcγRIIIb expresses HNA-1 antigens and is present in plasma.[20]

The gene frequencies of *HNA-1a*, *HNA-1b*, and *HNA-1c* vary widely among different racial groups. Among people of European ethnicity, the frequency of the gene encoding HNA-1a, *FCGR3B*1*, is between 0.30 and 0.37, and the frequency of the gene encoding HNA-1b, *FCGR3B*2*, is from 0.63 to 0.70.[21-25] In Japanese and Chinese populations, the *FCGR3B*1* gene frequency ranges from 0.60 to 0.66, and the *FCGR3B*2* gene frequency, from 0.30 to 0.33.[21,23-25] The frequency of the gene encoding HNA-1c, *FCGR3B*3*, also varies among racial groups. *FCGR3B*3* is expressed by neutrophils in 4% to 5% of

Table 6-1. Neutrophil-Specific Antigens

System	Alleles	Former Name	Location of Antigen	Gene	Comments
HNA-1	HNA-1a	NA1	FcγRIIIb	FCGR3B*1	Other polymorphisms in the HNA-1 system have been described.
HNA-1	HNA-1b	NA2	FcγRIIIb	FCGR3B*2	
HNA-1	HNA-1c	NA2	FcγRIIIb	FCGR3B*3	
HNA-2	HNA-2a	NB1	NB1gp	CD177*1	
HNA-3	HNA-3a	5b	Unknown	Unknown	Molecular basis of HNA-3a is not known.
HNA-4	HNA-4a	Mart[a]	α_M integrin, C3bi-receptor (CR3)	CD11B*1	
HNA-5	HNA-5a	Ond[a]	αL integrin, LFA-1	CD11A*1	

people of European ethnicity and 25% to 38% of people of African ethnicity.[26]

Although single nucleotide polymorphisms (SNPs) are responsible for many blood cell antigens, the molecular basis of HNA-1 polymorphisms is more complicated. The *FCGR3B*1* gene differs from the *FCGR3B*2* gene by five nucleotides in the coding region at positions 141, 147, 227, 277, and 349.[19,27-29] Four of the nucleotide changes result in changes in amino acid sequence between the HNA-1a and HNA-1b forms of the FcγRIIIb glycoprotein. The fifth polymorphism at 147 is silent. The glycosylation pattern of FcγRIIIb differs between HNA-1a and HNA-1b because of two nucleotide changes at bases 227 and 277. The HNA-1b form of FcγRIIIb has six *N*-linked glycosylation sites, and the HNA-1a form has four glycosylation sites.

The gene encoding HNA-1c, *FCGR3B*3*, is identical to *FCGR3B*2* except for a C to A substitution at nucleotide 266 that results in an alanine to aspartate change at amino acid 78 of FcγRIIIb.[18] In many cases, *FCGR3B*3* exists on the same chromosome with a second or duplicate *FCGR3B* gene.[30] One group has found that *FCGR3B*3* always exists in people of Danish ancestry as a duplicate gene in association with *FCGR3B*1*.[31] In other populations, however, duplicate *FCGR3B*3* genes have also been associated with *FCGR3B*1*.[31,32]

Several other sequence variations in *FCGR3B* have been described.[23,33] Most of these *FCGR3B* alleles have single-base substitutions involving one of the five single nucleotide polymorphisms that distinguish *FCGR3B*1* and *FCGR3B*2*. These unusual *FCGR3B* alleles are found more often in African Americans or African Brazilians than in people of European or Japanese ethnicity.[23,33]

Blood cells from patients with paroxysmal nocturnal hemoglobinuria lack the glycosyl-phosphatidylinositol (GPI)-linked glycoproteins, and their granulocytes express reduced amounts of FcγRIIIb and the HNA-1 antigens.[19] In addition, genetic deficiencies of granulocyte FcγRIIIb and HNA-1 antigens have also been reported. With an inherited deficiency of FcγRIIIb, the *FCGR3B* gene is deleted along with an adjacent gene,

FCGR2C.[34] Among people of European ethnicity, the incidence of individuals homozygous for *FCGR3B* deletion is about 0.1%.[35,36] However, among Africans and African Americans, the incidence is much higher. In one study, 3 of 126 Africans were found to be *FCGR3B* deficient,[26] and, in another, 1 of 53 were found to be *FCGR3B* deficient.[23] People with FcγRIIIb deficiency are healthy, but women with FcγRIIIb deficiency who become pregnant sometimes become alloimmunized and their children can experience alloimmune neonatal neutropenia.

HNA-2 Antigen System

The HNA-2 system has one allele, *HNA-2a*, which is located on the NB1 glycoprotein. *HNA-2a* was first described as NB1 by Lalezari et al in 1971.[37] Both *HNA-2a* and NB1 gp are encoded by the gene *CD177*, which is located on chromosome 19q13.3.[38,39] Historically, the gene encoding NB1 gp was cloned by Kissel and colleagues[38] and was called *NB1*. At the same time, a similar gene was identified by another group that was working to identify genes whose expression differed between neutrophils from patients with polycythemia vera (PV) and healthy subjects. The gene that was most strongly overexpressed in neutrophils from patients with PV was cloned, sequenced, and called *PRV-1*.[40] Both *NB1* and *PRV-1* encode a 437 amino acid GPI-anchored protein with 3 N-glycosylation sites that belongs to the uPAR/CD59/Ly6 snake toxin superfamily. The predicted amino acid sequences of the proteins encoded by *NB1* and *PRV-1* differ at only 4 amino acids.[38] Caruccio and colleagues have shown that *NB1* and *PRV-1* are alleles of the same gene, *CD177*, which is located on chromosome 19q13.3.[39]

CD177 encodes the NB1 gp, which is a 58 to 64 kDa GPI-anchored protein that is expressed only on neutrophils.[41] NB1 gp has been found to be an adhesion molecule. Sachs and colleagues have recently found that NB1 gp binds to platelet endothelial cell adhesion molecule-1 (PECAM-1, CD31).[42] PECAM-1 is expressed on both neutrophils and endothelial cells, and

PECAM-1/PECAM-1 interactions are important in the migration of neutrophils through endothelial cells. Interactions between NB1 gp and PECAM-1 are also involved with neutrophil-endothelial cell interactions and mediate neutrophil transendothelial cell migration.[42]

Neutrophils from 3% to 5% of a mixed-ethnicity population do not express HNA-2a. Serologic studies of neutrophils from such subjects suggest that their neutrophils lack the NB1 gp or at least a substantial portion of the molecule. Recently, Kissel and colleagues assessed *CD177* in two women who were HNA-2a-negative and who became alloimmunized to HNA-2a during pregnancy.[43] Both women had abnormally spliced *CD177* messenger ribonucleic acid (mRNA). None of the mRNA in these two women encoded for the complete NB1 gp. However, no specific *CD177* mutation or nucleotide deletion could be identified to account for the missplicing.

HNA-2a and NB1 gp are unique in that they are expressed on subpopulations of neutrophils. The mean proportion of neutrophils that express HNA-2a is approximately 50% and is slightly greater in females than in males.[44,45] Among the 4 polymorphic amino acids in NB1 gp, one has been found to affect the proportion of neutrophils that express NB1 gp. Caruccio and colleagues have found that a G42C polymorphism in *CD177* that causes an alanine to proline amino acid change in the protein's leader sequence results in reduced expression of NB1 gp.[46]

Several other factors affect neutrophil expression of HNA-2a and NB1 gp. The percentage of neutrophils that express HNA-2a is increased in pregnancy.[45] The expression of HNA-2a is greater in the second trimester than the first and is greatest in the third trimester.[47] The percentage of neutrophils that express HNA-2a is increased on neutrophil precursors, on peripheral blood neutrophils from healthy subjects given granulocyte colony-stimulating factors (G-CSF),[48,49] and on umbilical cord blood neutrophils.[50,51] The expression of HNA-2a is also increased on neutrophils from patients with severe bacterial infections.[49]

The expression of *CD177* mRNA by the HNA-2a-negative subpopulation of neutrophils found in people with a typical proportion of HNA-2a-positive neutrophils has also been studied. Although individuals whose neutrophils do not express any HNA-2a have abnormally spliced *CD177* mRNA, neutrophils that do not express HNA-2a in HNA-2a-positive individuals do not express any *CD177* mRNA.[52] The mechanism responsible for the lack of *CD177* transcription in these cells is not certain.

HNA-3, -4, and -5 Antigen Systems

Only one known polymorphism exists in each of the other three antigen systems, which are HNA-3, HNA-4, and HNA-5. The HNA-3 antigen system has one antigen, HNA-3a, that was previously known as 5b. HNA-3a is expressed by neutrophils, lymphocytes, platelets, endothelial cells, kidney, spleen, and placental cells. HNA-3a is expressed on neutrophils from approximately 90% of people of European ethnicity.[53] HNA-3a has a gene frequency of 0.66 and is located on a 70-kD to 95-kD neutrophil glycoprotein.[53] The gene encoding HNA-3a has not yet been cloned, and the nature and function of the 70-kD to 95-kD glycoprotein that carries HNA-3a are not known. Although the biologic role for this system has not been established, several cases of TRALI have been associated with the transfusion of plasma containing anti-HNA-3a.[13,54]

The HNA-4 and HNA-5 antigens are located on the β_2 integrins. The HNA-4a antigen was previously known as Mart[a]. HNA-4a was defined by an antibody in the sera of three non-transfused multiparous blood donors.[55] The antigen was shown to have autosomal-dominant inheritance and has a phenotype frequency of 99.1% in subjects of European ethnicity.[55] HNA-4a is located on the αM chain (CD11b) of the C3bi receptor (CR3) and is the result of a single nucleotide substitution of G to A at position 302.[56] The substitution would be predicted to result in an Arg-to-His polymorphism at amino acid 61.

A second polymorphism of the β_2 integrins, HNA-5a, was first described as Ond[a].[56,57] A multiply transfused man with aplastic anemia became alloimmunized to HNA-5a. HNA-5a was found to be expressed on the αL integrin unit, leukocyte function antigen-1 (LFA-1, or CD11a), and is the result of a G-to-C single nucleotide substitution at position 2446. This change predicts an amino acid change of Arg to Thr at amino acid 766.[56]

Neutrophil Antibody Detection

Several methods were established for antibody screening in the 1960s and 1970s, and these methods have remained largely unchanged (they are summarized in Table 6-2). Reagents and kits, although widely available for the detection of HLA antibodies, are not available for neutrophil antibody detection. Thus, screening for neutrophil antibodies remains technically challenging.

Most laboratories are using isolated neutrophils for antibody screening assays. The assays most commonly used to detect neutrophil antibodies are granulocyte agglutination (GA), granulocyte immunofluorescence (GIF) or flow cytometry, and monoclonal antibody immobilization of neutrophil antigens (MAINA). Antibodies are analyzed for specificity to specific antigens by testing against a panel of neutrophils from donors of known HNA phenotypes.

Neutrophil Isolation

Because neutrophils have a short life span, fresh neutrophils must be prepared daily for testing. For best results, neutrophils are isolated from the blood on the day that they are collected. Generally, neutrophils are isolated from anticoagulated whole blood using a two-step process. First, RBCs are separated from leukocytes by mixing hydroxyl ethyl starch, methyl cellulose, or dextran with the whole blood and allowing the RBCs to settle for 30 to 60 minutes. Then neutrophils are separated from the leukocytes using density gradient separation. Typically, ficoll-hypaque gradients of two different densities are used. After the

Table 6-2. Neutrophil Antibody Detection Methods

Assay	Source of Antigen	Antibodies Detected	Antibodies Not Detected
Granulocyte agglutination (GA)	Fresh neutrophils	All	None
Granulocyte immunofluorescence (GIF)	Fresh neutrophils	All	None
Monoclonal antibody immobilization of neutrophil antigens (MAINA)	Fresh neutrophils	HNA-1a, -1b, -1c, -2a, -4a, -5a	HNA-3a
Passive hemagglutination	Cryopreserved neutrophil extract	HNA-1a, -1b, -2a, -3a, -4a, -5a	HNA-1c
Cell lines	Transfected neutrophil genes	HNA-1a, -1b, -1c, -2a, -4a, -5a	HNA-3a

isolated neutrophils are washed, they are immediately used for testing.

Granulocyte Agglutination Assay

In the GA assay, antibodies cause neutrophils to actively agglutinate.[58] Isolated neutrophils and serum are incubated for 4 to 6 hours at 30 C. When neutrophil antibodies are present, neutrophils clump. The GA assay is very reliable but less sensitive than other assays. It can detect antibodies to HNA-1, -2, -3, -4, and -5 antigens, and it is the assay that can best identify antibodies specific for HNA-3a.[59]

Granulocyte Immunofluorescence Assay

In the GIF assay, antigen-antibody reactions are detected using fluorescence-conjugated secondary antibodies and a fluorescent microscope.[58] Before incubation with sera, isolated neutrophils are treated with 1% paraformaldehyde for 5 minutes at 20 C to 24 C to help prevent nonspecific binding of antibodies to neutrophil Fc receptors and to stabilize the cell membranes. Binding of antibodies to the neutrophils is detected with a fluorochrome-conjugated secondary antibody. When analyzed by fluorescent microscopy, the binding of antibodies in the test serum results in a uniform staining of the outside of the neutrophils. Strong reactions are readily distinguished, but considerable training is required to distinguish weak reactions from background staining, which can occur as a result of nonspecific binding of IgG to neutrophil Fc receptors. Testing for neutrophil antibodies with flow cytometry is performed using the same methods as used for the GIF assay except that neutrophils are evaluated with a flow cytometer rather than a fluorescent microscope. The flow cytometry assay has replaced the fluorescent microscope in most reference laboratories.

Monoclonal Antibody Immobilization of Neutrophil Antigens Assay

The MAINA assay allows the detection of antibodies to specific neutrophil membrane glycoproteins.[60-62] In this assay, neutrophils are incubated with test sera, washed, and incubated with a murine monoclonal antibody to a specific neutrophil glycoprotein. The neutrophils are then dissolved in a mild detergent. The soluble glycoprotein-monoclonal antibody complex is "captured" in a well with an antibody specific to mouse IgG fixed to the well bottom. An antibody specific to human IgG conjugated to alkaline phosphatase is added, followed by a substrate, and the reaction is detected with a spectrophotometer. Alternatively, the reactions can be detected by chemiluminescence.

The MAINA assay can be used to detect antibodies specific to HNA-1a, -1b, and -1c on FcγRIIIb (CD16); HNA-2a on NB1 gp (CD177); HNA-4a on complement component C3bi receptor (CR3 or CD11b); and HNA-5a on leukocyte function antigen-1 (LFA-1 or CD11a). The use of neutrophils from panels of donors with known HNA-1 phenotypes allows the identification of antibodies specific to HNA-1a, -1b, and -1c. In addition, antibodies are sometimes detected that are directed toward FcγRIIIb but are not specific to HNA-1a, -1b, or -1c. Because the neutrophil membrane molecule carrying HNA-3a has not yet been described, a monoclonal antibody is not available to test for antibodies to HNA-3a in the MAINA assay. The MAINA assay permits the recognition of antibodies to specific neutrophil glycoproteins even when antibodies to HLA antigens are present.

Mixed Passive Agglutination

The mixed passive agglutination assay uses a granulocyte antigen preparation rather than intact granulocytes for antibody screening.[63,64] This assay allows granulocyte testing trays to be prepared in large batches and frozen until testing. Antigens are extracted from isolated neutrophils using 3% sucrose. The neutrophil extract is used to coat U-bottom Terasaki plates. Sera to be tested are incubated with neutrophil extract in wells for 3 hours at 22 C. Antibody binding is detected using sheep erythrocytes coated with antihuman IgG. The antigen-coated plates can be prepared and stored for at least 1 year at −80 C.

Araki and colleagues found that the assay detected antibodies to HNA-1a, -1b, -2a, and -3a.[63] Han and colleagues have confirmed that this assay can detect antibodies to HNA-1a, -1b, and -2a, and they found that it detected antibodies to HNA-4a and -5a antigens.[64] This test is not commercially available and reagents must be prepared by the laboratory performing the testing.

Expression of Antigens in Cell Lines

Another approach to test for neutrophil antibodies is to transfect K562 cells with the genes encoding neutrophil antigens HNA-1a, -1b, and -2a.[65] In this assay, serum or plasma to be tested for neutrophil antibodies is incubated with the transfected K562 cells, and flow cytometry is used to assess antibody reactivity. However, the molecular basis of HNA-3a is not known, and this approach cannot be used to test for antibodies to this antigen.

Strategy for Antibody Detection

Most laboratories screen for neutrophil antibodies by testing serum against panels of granulocytes in GA, GIF, or flow cytometry assays. Because HLA Class I antibodies can react with neutrophils in GA, GIF, and flow cytometry assays, if HLA Class I antibodies are present in a reactive sample, the sample must be tested in the MAINA or a similar assay to determine if both HLA Class I and neutrophil-specific antibodies are present. Because the MAINA assay sometimes identifies antibodies that cannot be detected in other assays, some laboratories test all serum samples in MAINA assays. Serum can also be tested against cell lines that express neutrophil antigens, but not HLA Class I antigens. Another alternative to determine if an antibody is specific to neutrophil or HLA Class I antigens is to adsorb that reactive sample with platelets and to repeat the testing. Because platelets express HLA Class I antigens but not neutrophil-specific antigens, platelet adsorption selectively removes antibodies to HLA Class I antigens.

Typing of Neutrophil Antigens

Traditionally, neutrophil-specific antigens were identified and phenotyped with techniques that used alloantibodies and isolated leukocytes. When possible, serologic typing is being replaced by genotyping for several reasons. Alloantibodies that come from the sera of alloimmunized patients or donors are difficult to obtain, and typing with alloantibodies is less precise than molecular typing. Phenotyping assays also require working with fresh whole blood samples, and granulocytes must be isolated from red cells and other leukocytes. In contrast, genotyping methods do not require fresh blood samples or the separation of leukocytes from other blood cells. Another advantage to genotyping is that DNA can be easily stored for many months before testing, whereas isolated granulocytes must be tested within a day of collection.

Table 6-3 summarizes neutrophil antigen detection methods.

Phenotyping Neutrophil Antigens

Traditionally, neutrophil antigen phenotyping has been performed using human alloantibodies in the GA or GIF assays. Alloantibodies to HLA-1a, -1b, -2a, and -3a are available, but antibodies to HNA-1c, -4a, and -5a are difficult to obtain. Monoclonal antibodies specific to HNA-1a, -1b, and -2a have been described; they are commercially available and have been used to phenotype neutrophils using flow cytometry. Granulocyte

---

Table 6-3. Neutrophil Antigen Detection Methods

Assay	Comments
Granulocyte agglutina-tion (GA)	Uses alloantibodies of known specificity; best method for detecting HNA-3a.
Granulocyte immunoflu-orescence (GIF)	Monoclonal antibodies specific for HNA-1a, -1b, and -2a are available.
Genotyping	A commercial kit is available for HNA-1a, -1b, and -1c typing; genotyping cannot be performed for HNA-2a and HNA-3a.

---

phenotyping with monoclonal antibodies and flow cytometry is faster and easier than phenotyping with alloantibodies. Phenotyping with alloantibodies requires the isolation of neutrophils, whereas phenotyping with monoclonal antibodies can be performed using whole blood instead of isolated neutrophils.

Genotyping Neutrophil Antigens

Genotyping assays for HNA-1a, -1b, -1c, -4a, and -5a have been developed. The characterization of the genes encoding the HNA-1 antigens has allowed for the development of genotyping assays for these antigens.[21,22,26] Genotyping for *FCGR3B* alleles is complicated by the high degree of homology between *FCGR3B* and the gene that encodes FcγRIIIa, *FCGR3A*. Among the five nucleotides that differ between *FCGR3B*1* and *FCGR3B*2*, *FCGR3A* is the same as *FCGR3B*1* at three nucleotides and the same as *FCGR3B*2* at two nucleotides. As a result, most laboratories use polymerase chain reaction (PCR) and sequence-specific primers (SSPs) to distinguish *FCGR3B* alleles. A unique set of primers is used to amplify each of the three alleles. A commercial PCR-SSP kit is available for genotyping

HNA-1a, -1b, and -1c. Methods to genotype neutrophil antigens HNA-4a and HNA-5a have been described.[56] A PCR-SSP method is being used to type HNA-4a.[66] HNA-5a can be typed using either a PCR-SSP method[67] or a PCR restriction fragment length polymorphism method.[68]

Although the molecular basis of HNA-2a has been described, HNA-2a genotyping methods are not available. The HNA-2a-negative phenotype is the result of *CD177* mRNA splicing defects.[43] The *CD177* mRNA from people with HNA-2a-negative neutrophils contains additional sequences of varying length that are homologous to *CD177* intron sequences. However, no mutations have been detected in the *CD177* introns or exons from people with HNA-2a-negative neutrophils. It may be possible to distinguish the HNA-2a-positive and -negative phenotypes by analyzing neutrophil *CD177* mRNA for accessory sequences. However, working with mRNA is much more difficult than working with DNA, and mRNA is not being routinely analyzed to assess HNA-2a antigen expression. Because the gene encoding HNA-3a has not been identified, no genotyping assay is available for this antigen.

Evaluation of Patients and Donors Involved in TRALI

When a patient experiences TRALI or a severe pulmonary transfusion reaction, a possible role for leukocyte antibodies in the transfusion reaction should be investigated. Even if the patient does not experience a reaction severe enough to meet the criteria for TRALI, a leukocyte antibody investigation may be indicated—especially if the patient becomes neutropenic.[69]

The first step in the investigation is to test all associated blood donors for leukocyte antibodies. Serum is generally the preferred sample. Most laboratories have not validated their assays with segments or portions of Fresh Frozen Plasma (FFP) or platelets, but if these samples are free from contaminating cells and debris, presumably they should be suitable for testing. Because plasma from RBCs stored in additive solutions is diluted significantly, the results of testing segments or supernatants from these components would likely differ considerably from the results of testing the donor's serum. The evaluation should not be restricted to women or multiparous women, and testing should not be limited to HLA antibodies. All male and female donors should be tested for antibodies to both neutrophil and HLA antibodies. HLA antibody testing should include both HLA Class I and Class II antibodies. It may be helpful to type recipients who are shown to have been transfused with neutrophil antibodies for neutrophil antigens and those transfused with HLA antibodies for HLA antigens.

The need to test transfusion recipients who develop TRALI for leukocyte antibodies is controversial because of the fact that many cellular blood components are leukocyte reduced. However, granulocyte transfusion recipients are the exception. Recipients of granulocyte concentrates who experience pulmonary transfusion reactions or TRALI should be tested for both neutrophil and HLA antibodies.

Deferring Donors with Neutrophil Antibodies

It is widely accepted that both HLA and neutrophil-specific antibodies with a defined antigen specificity (ie, antibodies directed to a known neutrophil antigen such as HNA-1a, -1b, -2a, or -3a) are responsible for febrile transfusion reactions that occur following the transfusion of leukocyte-containing blood components. However, the role of leukocyte antibodies in TRALI is complex. There have been many cases of reports that link the transfusion of neutrophil-specific and HLA antibodies to ALI, but often the transfusion of leukocyte antibodies does not result in a transfusion reaction. Nevertheless, because the incidence of neutrophil-specific antibodies in healthy blood donors is low, and because the probability of a transfusion reaction is high when a component with neutrophil-specific antibodies such as HNA-2a[69] or HNA-3a[13,70] is transfused, at most centers, donors with neutrophil-specific antibodies to a defined antigen are deferred from further donations.

Although neutrophil-specific antibodies are often directed toward a defined antigen such as HNA-1a, -1b, -2a, or -3a, in most cases neutrophil-specific antibodies are not directed toward one of these defined antigens—ie, neutrophil antibodies are found on a neutrophil screening assay but no defined antigen specificity is found on further testing. Possible explanations for such a reaction pattern include an antibody to a currently undefined antigen specificity, a cross-reactive antibody, or a false-positive result. Because the pathophysiologic significance of neutrophil antibodies that lack specificity to a described antigen is uncertain, there is no consensus about the appropriate action to take if a donor associated with TRALI has such an antibody. The most conservative approach would be to defer such a donor from all future donation, the intermediate approach would be to divert the donor into low plasma-volume component donations (ie, not FFP or platelet apheresis), and the least conservative approach would be to allow such a donor to continue donating.

Conclusion

Several assays are available to determine neutrophil antigen phenotypes and to detect neutrophil antibodies. Either monoclonal antibodies specific for neutrophil antigens or genotyping assays are available for all antigens except HNA-3a. The traditional cellular assays (ie, GA, GIF, and MAINA) remain the most commonly used assays to test for neutrophil antibodies. Solid-phase assays and assays that make use of proteins carrying neutrophil-specific antigens expressed in cell lines have been described but are not widely used.

References

1. Brittingham TE. Immunologic studies on leukocytes. Vox Sang 1957;2:242-8.
2. King KE, Shirey RS, Thoman SK, et al. Universal leukoreduction decreases the incidence of febrile nonhemolytic transfusion reactions to RBCs. Transfusion 2004;44:25-9.
3. Paglino JC, Pomper GJ, Fisch GS, et al. Reduction of febrile but not allergic reactions to RBCs and platelets after conversion to universal prestorage leukoreduction. Transfusion 2004;44:16-24.
4. Yazer MH, Podlosky L, Clarke G, Nahirniak S. The effect of prestorage WBC reduction on the rates of febrile nonhemolytic transfusion reactions to platelet concentrates and RBC. Transfusion 2004;44:10-15.
5. Stroncek DF, Shapiro RS, Filipovich AH, et al. Prolonged neutropenia resulting from antibodies to neutrophil-specific antigen NB1 following marrow transplantation. Transfusion 1993;33:158-63.
6. Stroncek DF, Leonard K, Eiber G, et al. Alloimmunization after granulocyte transfusions. Transfusion 1996;36:1009-15.
7. Sachs UJ, Bux J. TRALI after the transfusion of cross-match-positive granulocytes. Transfusion 2003;43:1683-6.
8. Philipps E, Fleischner FG. Pulmonary edema in the course of a blood transfusion without overloading the circulation. Dis Chest 1966;50:619-23.
9. Ward HN, Lipscomb TS, Cawley LP. Pulmonary hypersensitivity reaction after blood transfusion. Arch Intern Med 1968;122:362-6.
10. Popovsky MA, Abel MD, Moore SB. Transfusion-related acute lung injury associated with passive transfer of antileukocyte antibodies. Am Rev Respir Dis 1983;128:185-9.
11. Yomtovian R, Kline W, Press C, et al. Severe pulmonary hypersensitivity associated with passive transfusion of a neutrophil-specific antibody. Lancet 1984;1:244-6.
12. Bux J, Becker F, Seeger W, et al. Transfusion-related acute lung injury due to HLA-A2-specific antibodies in recipient and NB1-specific antibodies in donor blood. Br J Haematol 1996;93:707-13.
13. Kopko PM, Marshall CS, MacKenzie MR, et al. Transfusion-related acute lung injury: Report of a clinical look-back investigation. JAMA 2002;287:1968-71.
14. Davoren A, Curtis BR, Shulman IA, et al. TRALI due to granulocyte-agglutinating human neutrophil antigen-3a (5b) alloantibodies in donor plasma: A report of 2 fatalities. Transfusion 2003;43:641-5.
15. Bux J. ISBT Working Party on Platelet and Granulocyte Serology, Granulocyte Antigen Working Party. International Society of Blood Transfusion. Nomenclature of granulocyte alloantigens. Transfusion 1999;39:662-3.
16. Lalezari P, Bernard GE. An isologous antigen-antibody reaction with human neutrophils, related to neonatal neutropenia. J Clin Invest 1966;45:1741-50.
17. Boxer LA, Yokoyama M, Lalezari P. Isoimmune neonatal neutropenia. J Pediatr 1972;80:783-7.
18. Bux J, Stein EL, Bierling P, et al. Characterization of a new alloantigen (SH) on the human neutrophil Fc gamma receptor IIIb. Blood 1997;89:1027-34.

19. Huizinga TW, Kleijer M, Tetteroo PA, et al. Biallelic neutrophil Na-antigen system is associated with a polymorphism on the phospho-inositol-linked Fc gamma receptor III (CD16). Blood 1990;75:213-17.

20. Huizinga TW, de Haas M, Kleijer M, et al. Soluble Fc gamma receptor III in human plasma originates from release by neutrophils. J Clin Invest 1990;86: 416-23.

21. Hessner MJ, Curtis BR, Endean DJ, et al. Determination of neutrophil antigen gene frequencies in five ethnic groups by polymerase chain reaction with sequence-specific primers. Transfusion 1996;36:895-9.

22. Bux J, Stein EL, Santoso S, et al. NA gene frequencies in the German population, determined by polymerase chain reaction with sequence-specific primers. Transfusion 1995;35:54-7.

23. Matsuo K, Procter J, Stroncek D. Variations in genes encoding neutrophil antigens NA1 and NA2. Transfusion 2000;40:645-53.

24. Lin M, Chen CC, Wang CL, et al. Frequencies of neutrophil-specific antigens among Chinese in Taiwan. Vox Sang 1994;66:247.

25. Ohto H, Matsuo Y. Neutrophil-specific antigens and gene frequencies in Japanese (letter). Transfusion 1989;29:654.

26. Kissel K, Hofmann C, Gittinger FS, et al. HNA-1a, HNA-1b, and HNA-1c (NA1, NA2, SH) frequencies in African and American Blacks and in Chinese. Tissue Antigens 2000;56:143-8.

27. Trounstine ML, Peltz GA, Yssel H, et al. Reactivity of cloned, expressed human Fc gamma RIII isoforms with monoclonal antibodies which distinguish cell-type-specific and allelic forms of Fc gamma RIII. Int Immunol 1990;2:303-10.

28. Ravetch JV, Perussia B. Alternative membrane forms of Fc gamma RIII(CD16) on human natural killer cells and neutrophils. Cell type-specific expression of two genes that differ in single nucleotide substitutions. J Exp Med 1989;170: 481-97.

29. Ory PA, Clark MR, Kwoh EE, et al. Sequences of complementary DNAs that encode the NA1 and NA2 forms of Fc receptor III on human neutrophils. J Clin Invest 1989;84:1688-91.

30. Koene HR, Kleijer M, Roos D, et al. Fc gamma RIIIB gene duplication: Evidence for presence and expression of three distinct Fc gamma RIIIB genes in NA(1+,2+)SH(+) individuals. Blood 1998;91:673-9.

31. Steffensen R, Gulen T, Varming K, et al. FcgammaRIIIB polymorphism: Evidence that NA1/NA2 and SH are located in two closely linked loci and that the SH allele is linked to the NA1 allele in the Danish population. Transfusion 1999;39:593-8.

32. Guz K, Brojer E, Zupanska B. Implications of NA1/NA2 and SH genotyping results in the Polish population with regard to the new nomenclature of granulocyte alloantigens. Transfusion 2000;40:490-1.

33. Covas DT, Kashima S, Guerreiro JF, et al. Variation in the FcgammaR3B gene among distinct Brazilian populations. Tissue Antigens 2005;65:178-82.

34. de Haas M, Kleijer M, van Zwieten R, et al. Neutrophil Fc gamma RIIIb deficiency, nature, and clinical consequences: A study of 21 individuals from 14 families. Blood 1995;86:2403-13.

35. Muniz-Diaz E, Madoz P, de la Calle MO, et al. The polymorphonuclear neutrophil Fc gamma RIIIb deficiency is more frequent than hitherto assumed. Blood 1995;86:3999.

36. Fromont P, Bettaieb A, Skouri H, et al. Frequency of the polymorphonuclear neutrophil Fc gamma receptor III deficiency in the French population and its involvement in the development of neonatal alloimmune neutropenia. Blood 1992;79:2131-4.

37. Lalezari P, Murphy GB, Allen FH Jr. NB1, a new neutrophil-specific antigen involved in the pathogenesis of neonatal neutropenia. J Clin Invest 1971;50:1108-15.

38. Kissel K, Santoso S, Hofmann C, et al. Molecular basis of the neutrophil glycoprotein NB1 (CD177) involved in the pathogenesis of immune neutropenias and transfusion reactions. Eur J Immunol 2001;31:1301-9.

39. Caruccio L, Bettinotti M, Director-Myska AE, et al. The gene overexpressed in polycythemia rubra vera, PRV-1, and the gene encoding a neutrophil alloantigen, NB1, are alleles of a single gene, CD177, in chromosome band 19q13.31. Transfusion 2006;46:441-7.

40. Temerinac S, Klippel S, Strunck E, et al. Cloning of PRV-1, a novel member of the uPAR receptor superfamily, which is overexpressed in polycythemia rubra vera. Blood 2000;95:2569-76.

41. Stroncek DF, Skubitz KM, McCullough JJ. Biochemical characterization of the neutrophil-specific antigen NB1. Blood 1990;75:744-55.

42. Sachs UJ, Andrei-Selmer CL, Maniar A, et al. The neutrophil-specific antigen CD177 is a counter-receptor for platelet endothelial cell adhesion molecule-1 (CD31). J Biol Chem 2007;282:23603-12.

43. Kissel K, Scheffler S, Kerowgan M, et al. Molecular basis of NB1 (HNA-2a, CD177) deficiency. Blood 2002;99:4231-3.

44. Matsuo K, Lin A, Procter JL, et al. Variations in the expression of granulocyte antigen NB1. Transfusion 2000;40:654-62.

45. Caruccio L, Bettinotti M, Matsuo K, et al. Expression of human neutrophil antigen-2a (NB1) is increased in pregnancy. Transfusion 2003;43:357-63.

46. Caruccio L, Walkovich K, Bettinotti M, et al. CD177 polymorphisms: Correlation between high-frequency single nucleotide polymorphisms and neutrophil surface protein expression. Transfusion 2004;44:77-82.

47. Taniguchi K, Nagata H, Katsuki T, et al. Significance of human neutrophil antigen-2a (NB1) expression and neutrophil number in pregnancy. Transfusion 2004;44:581-5.

48. Stroncek DF, Jaszcz W, Herr GP, et al. Expression of neutrophil antigens after 10 days of granulocyte-colony-stimulating factor. Transfusion 1998;38:663-8.

49. Gohring K, Wolff J, Doppl W, et al. Neutrophil CD177 (NB1 gp, HNA-2a) expression is increased in severe bacterial infections and polycythaemia vera. Br J Haematol 2004;126:252-4.

50. Stroncek DF, Shankar R, Litz C, et al. The expression of the NB1 antigen on myeloid precursors and neutrophils from children and umbilical cords. Transfus Med 1998;8:119-23.

51. Wolff JC, Goehring K, Heckmann M, et al. Sex-dependent up regulation of CD177-specific mRNA expression in cord blood due to different stimuli. Transfusion 2006;46:132-6.

52. Wolff J, Brendel C, Fink L, et al. Lack of NB1 GP (CD177/HNA-2a) gene transcription in NB1 GP-neutrophils from NB1 GP-expressing individuals and association of low expression with NB1 gene polymorphisms. Blood 2003;102: 731-3.

53. de Haas M, Muniz-Diaz E, Alonso LG, et al. Neutrophil antigen 5b is carried by a protein, migrating from 70 to 95 kDa, and may be involved in neonatal alloimmune neutropenia. Transfusion 2000;40:222-7.

54. Nordhagen R, Conradi M, Dromtorp SM. Pulmonary reaction associated with transfusion of plasma containing anti-5b. Vox Sang 1986;51:102-7.

55. Kline WE, Press C, Clay M, et al. Three sera defining a new granulocyte-monocyte-T-lymphocyte antigen. Vox Sang 1986;50:181-6.

56. Simsek S, van der Schoot CE, Daams M, et al. Molecular characterization of antigenic polymorphisms (Ond(a) and Mart(a)) of the beta 2 family recognized by human leukocyte alloantisera. Blood 1996;88:1350-8.

57. Decary F, Verheugt FW, Helden-Henningheim L, et al. Recognition of a non-HLA-ABC antigen present on B and T lymphocytes and monocytes only detectable with the indirect immunofluorescence test. Vox Sang 1979;36:150-8.

58. McCullough J, Clay M, Press C, Kline W. Granulocyte serology: A clinical and laboratory guide. Chicago: American Society of Clinical Pathologists Press, 1988.

59. Bux J, Chapman J. Report on the second international granulocyte serology workshop. Transfusion 1997;37:977-83.

60. Bux J, Kober B, Kiefel V, et al. Analysis of granulocyte-reactive antibodies using an immunoassay based upon monoclonal-antibody-specific immobilization of granulocyte antigens. Transfus Med 1993;3:157-62.

61. Metcalfe P, Waters AH. Location of the granulocyte-specific antigen LAN on the Fc-receptor III. Transfus Med 1992;2:283-7.

62. Nishimura M, Takanashi M, Okazaki H, et al. Detection of anti-CD32 alloantibody in donor plasma implicated in development of transfusion-related acute lung injury. Cell Biochem Funct 2005;25:179-83.

63. Araki N, Nose Y, Kohsaki M, et al. Anti-granulocyte antibody screening with extracted granulocyte antigens by a micro-mixed passive hemagglutination method. Vox Sang 1999;77:44-51.

64. Han TH, Chey MJ, Han KS. Granulocyte antibodies in Korean neonates with neutropenia. J Korean Med Sci 2006;21:627-32.

65. Yasui K, Miyazaki T, Matsuyama N, et al. Establishment of cell lines stably expressing HNA-1a, -1b, and -2a antigen with low background reactivity in flow cytometric analysis. Transfusion 2007;47:478-85.

66. Clague HD, Fung YL, Minchinton RM. Human neutrophil antigen-4a gene frequencies in an Australian population, determined by a new polymerase chain reaction method using sequence-specific primers. Transfus Med 2003;13:149-52.

67. Sachs UJ, Reil A, Bauer C, et al. Genotyping of human neutrophil antigen-5a (Ond). Transfus Med 2005;15:115-17.

68. Cardone JD, Bordin JO, Chiba AK, et al. Gene frequencies of the HNA-4a and -5a neutrophil antigens in Brazilian persons and a new polymerase chain reaction-restriction fragment length polymorphism method for HNA-5a genotyping. Transfusion 2006;46:1515-20.

69. Fadeyi EA, Los Angeles MM, Wayne AS, et al. The transfusion of neutrophil-specific antibodies causes leukopenia and a broad spectrum of pulmonary reactions. Transfusion 2007;47:545-50.

70. Muniz M, Sheldon S, Schuller RM, et al. Patient-specific transfusion-related acute lung injury. Vox Sang 2008;94:70-3.

In: Kleinman S, Popovsky MA, eds.
TRALI: Mechanisms, Management, and Prevention
Bethesda, MD: AABB Press, 2008

7

UK Hemovigilance and the Preferential Use of Male-Donor Plasma

CATHERINE E. CHAPMAN, BSc, MD, FRCP, FRCPATH, AND LORNA M. WILLIAMSON, BSc, MD, FRCP, FRCPATH

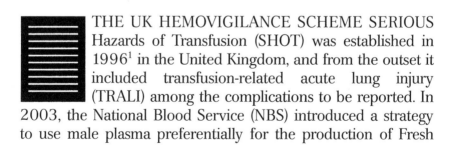 THE UK HEMOVIGILANCE SCHEME SERIOUS Hazards of Transfusion (SHOT) was established in 1996[1] in the United Kingdom, and from the outset it included transfusion-related acute lung injury (TRALI) among the complications to be reported. In 2003, the National Blood Service (NBS) introduced a strategy to use male plasma preferentially for the production of Fresh

Catherine E. Chapman, BSc, MD, FRCP, FRCPath, Consultant in Transfusion Medicine, National Health Service Blood and Transplant (Newcastle Blood Centre), Newcastle, United Kingdom, and Lorna M. Williamson, BSc, MD, FRCP, FRCPath, Reader in Transfusion Medicine, University of Cambridge, and Medical Director, National Health Service Blood and Transplant, Cambridge, United Kingdom
Funding provided by the UK Blood Services.

Frozen Plasma (FFP) and the suspension of buffy-coat-derived pooled platelets. This chapter describes 195 TRALI cases reported to SHOT from 1996 to 2006, and it assesses the effect of the preferentially male plasma policy.

Overview

SHOT accepts reports of serious adverse events related to labile blood components issued by the four UK Blood Transfusion Services. Investigation of a suspected TRALI case is the responsibility of the hospital and the NBS, with results made available to SHOT. Until 2006, participation in SHOT was voluntary but was endorsed by the Department of Health.

From 1996 to 2005, TRALI cases were defined by SHOT as "acute dyspnoea with hypoxia and bilateral pulmonary infiltrates occurring during or in the 24 hours after transfusion, with no other apparent cause," with no requirement for any specific serologic findings. In 2006, on the basis of previous findings and the recommendations of the Canadian Consensus Conference,[2] SHOT reduced the time frame from 24 hours to 6 hours.[3] In 1999, SHOT introduced a system to assess the likelihood of the reported cases actually being TRALI on the basis of fluid balance, the presence of cardiac failure, other risk factors for acute lung injury (ALI), and donor/patient leukocyte serology. After review by 2 SHOT clinicians, including an intensivist beginning in 2004, cases were allocated as follows:

- **Highly likely:** A convincing clinical picture and positive serology existed (donor or patient leukocyte antibodies corresponding with recipient/donor antigens or a positive leukocyte crossmatch, or both).
- **Probable:** Either a less convincing history and positive serology existed *or* a good history and less convincing or absent serology.
- **Possible:** The clinical picture and/or serology was compatible with TRALI, but other causes could not be excluded.

- **Unlikely:** The clinical picture and serology were not supportive of the diagnosis.

Between 1996 and 2006, 218 complete reports of suspected TRALI were received by SHOT. Of these, 23 were subsequently withdrawn because the reporter considered another diagnosis more likely, leaving 195 cases for analysis. As shown in Fig 7-1, TRALI reports increased from 9 in 1996/1997 to a peak of 36 in 2003, with subsequent decreases at least partly resulting from the male plasma policy. Criteria for assessing the likelihood of a case being TRALI, on the basis of clinical features and serology, were introduced in 1999. Of the subsequent 156 cases, 51 were assessed as highly likely, 25 as probable, 42 as possible, and 38 cases as unlikely. Patient ages ranged from 26 days to 83 years, with a median of 56 years. Children accounted for 20 cases (9.7%). There was no significant gender bias.

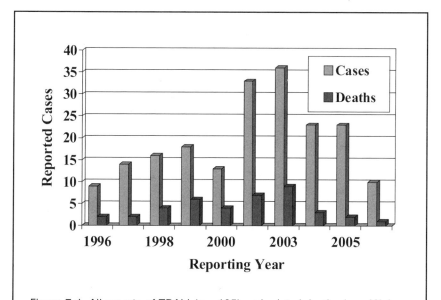

Figure 7-1. All reports of TRALI (n = 195) and related deaths (n = 40) from 1996 to 2006, inclusive. Reporting years from 1996 to 2000 each cover 12 months from October 1 through September 30. The 2001 report covers 15 months from October 1, 2001 through December 31, 2002; 2003 and subsequent year reports cover calendar years.

The most frequent clinical specialties represented were hematology and oncology combined (36%) and surgery (36%). Cardiac surgery had occurred in 18 cases (10%), 9 cases (5%) were associated with the use of FFP to reverse warfarin, and a further 9 cases (5%) were associated with plasma exchange with FFP for thrombotic thrombocytopenic purpura (TTP).

The Data

Clinical Features and Outcomes

By definition, all patients had acute dyspnea, hypoxia, and bilateral pulmonary infiltrates. Fever and hypotension also existed in 37% and 52% of cases, respectively, but no difference existed in the incidence of these secondary features between highly likely or probable cases and between those considered possible or unlikely. Of 151 cases up to 2005, 139 (92%) occurred either during or within 6 hours of transfusion, 7 (5%) between 6 and 12 hours of transfusion, and 5 (3%) between 12 and 24 hours of transfusion, with similar percentages for the highly likely or probable cases.

Of the 195 cases, 143 (73%) required admission to intensive therapy units (ITUs) or were already in ITUs when the reaction occurred, with 88 (45%) requiring mechanical ventilation. Of the 195, 40 deaths (21%) occurred in which TRALI was considered at least a contributory factor, with similar percentages for highly likely or probable and for possible or unlikely cases. Long-term morbidity was reported in 10 cases (5%), of which 6 had impaired respiratory function, and 1 also had cerebral damage associated with prolonged mechanical ventilation (>110 days). No details of the morbidity suffered were reported for 2 cases but 1 had been mechanically ventilated for >50 days. The final case with long-term morbidity had recovered from the acute respiratory symptoms within 24 hours but was found to have suffered a concomitant myocardial infarction that was attributed to the TRALI reaction. The remaining 145 of 195 cases (74%) either made a full recovery or died of an unrelated cause.

Serologic Findings

From 2000 onward, most patients and implicated donors were well investigated for leukocyte antibodies. Donors were recalled to give fresh samples, which gave less nonspecific reactivity in immunofluorescence assays than frozen archived samples. All female donors and previously transfused males were investigated. If there were no antibodies that matched donor antigens found in either of these donor groups, and if there was good clinical evidence for TRALI, then the donor investigation was extended to untransfused male donors. Samples were screened for HLA Class I antibodies (and HLA Class II, beginning in 2001) by enzyme-linked immunosorbent assay (ELISA) and for Class I also by the microlymphocytotoxicity test (LCT). One Lambda LABScreen (One Lambda, Canoga Park, CA) replaced both ELISA and LCT in 2005. HNA antibody screening was performed with the granulocyte immunofluorescence test (GIFT), lymphocyte immunofluorescence test (LIFT), and granulocyte chemiluminescence test using cells obtained from a panel of typed donors.[4] If a leukocyte antibody with a defined specificity was found in a donor, genotyping or phenotyping of the recipient sample was performed to establish whether the cognate antigen was present. If nonspecific HLA or granulocyte antibodies were detected, a flow-cytometric crossmatch (GIFT/ LIFT) was undertaken.

Between 1996 and 1999, 43 of 57 (75%) cases either had no results or had inconclusive findings. From 2000 to 2006, donor antibodies recognizing a cognate antigen in the patient were identified in 62 of 96 completely investigated cases (65%), with the remaining 34 cases (35%) having no donor antibodies detected.

Antibodies matched a patient HLA Class I antigen in 12 donors (19%), matched an HLA Class II antigen in 25 donors (41%), and matched both in 13 (21%), meaning that HLA Class

II antibodies were implicated in 62% of antibody-positive cases. The most common antibody specificities were HLA Class II antigens DR52 and DR4, being found in 13 (18%) and 12 (16%) cases, respectively, followed by HLA-A2 in 10 cases (13%). In 18 cases (24%), more than one antibody with cognate antigen specificity (termed a "concordant antibody") was found. Granulocyte-specific antibodies recognizing a cognate patient antigen were found in 9 of 62 cases (14%), with HNA-1a the most frequent (5 cases). Of the 9 cases, only 1 also had a donor with cognate HLA antibodies. It is significant that all donors found to have concordant HLA or granulocyte antibodies were female.

HLA antibodies were found in 30 of 114 patients tested (15%), and granulocyte antibodies were found in 1. Antibody concordance with donor antigens was not fully assessed in most patients and was established in only 3 cases, all of which occurred after the introduction of universal leukocyte reduction.

Implicated Components and Their Relationship to Positive Donor Serology

In 2003, a review of all TRALI reports since 1996 was carried out. As shown in Table 7-1, the risk per component for TRALI was 6.86 times higher for FFP/cryosupernatant than for red cells [95% confidence interval (CI), 4.2-11.2], and it was 8.16 times higher for platelets than for red cells (95% CI, 4.91-13.37). These values show statistical significance, unlike the relative risk from cryoprecipitate over red cells, which was 1.76 (0.42-7.32). Moreover, as shown in Table 7-2, in TRALI cases where red cells had been implicated, exposure to an antibody-positive female donor was no greater than expected ($p = 0.08$). In contrast, recipients in whom FFP or platelets were the implicated component had a much greater than expected exposure to an antibody-positive female donor ($p < 0.0001$). The "expected" figure was based on a previous study that demonstrated HLA antibodies in 15% of female donors.[5] A separate study has demonstrated that each transfusion episode consists of a median of 3 donor exposures [A Wells, Epidemiology and Survival

Table 7-1. Implicated Components in All TRALI Reports, 1996-2003, and Relative Risk of TRALI from Different Components

	Red Cells	Cryopre-cipitate	FFP/Cryosuper-natant	Platelets
TRALI cases in which compo-nent was impli-cated	33	2	31	27
Components issued (000s)	18,370	634	2515	1842
Risk/component issued*	1:556,000	1:317,000	1:81,000	1:68,000
Relative risk com-pared to red cells (95% CI)	—	1.76 (0.42-7.32)	6.86 (4.2-11.2)[†]	8.16 (4.91-13.37)[†]

*To nearest thousand.
[†]Statistically significant because 95% confidence interval does not contain 1.

of Transfusion Recipients (EASTR) study, unpublished observations]. Therefore, of 33 transfusion episodes from a total of 100 donors, 7 episodes (20%) would be expected to include a component from an HLA antibody-positive female donor by chance.

Implementation and Effect of the Preferentially Male Plasma Policy for FFP and Suspension of Platelet Pools

In October 2003, on the basis of the previous data, NBS introduced a policy to make FFP preferentially from male donors, because their incidence of HLA and HNA antibodies is low,[5] and to suspend buffy-coat-derived platelet pools in male plasma.

Table 7-2. Relationship between Implicated Component, Serology, and Donor Gender in 74 Fully Investigated Cases of TRALI, 1998-2003

	Red Cells	FFP/Platelets
All cases	18	56
Cases with antibody-positive donor	6	44
Proportion of all cases in which exposure to antibody-positive donor was expected*	0.2	0.2
Proportion of all cases in which exposure to antibody-positive donor was observed (95% CI)	0.33 (0.12-0.55)[†]	0.79 (0.68-0.89)[‡]
Gender of antibody-positive donors	3/3 female[§]	34/34 female[§]
Gender of donors with antibodies matching patient antigens or a positive crossmatch	2/2 female	29/29 female

*Based on MacLennan et al.[5]
[†]$p = 0.08$.
[‡]$p < 0.0001$.
[§]In other cases, donor gender was not identified from the investigating laboratory.
FFP = Fresh Frozen Plasma; CI = confidence interval.

To maintain supplies, NBS did not withdraw FFP from female donors that was in storage, but it was gradually phased out. Blood collection staff marked whole blood donations as "M" or "F," and, at the processing center, the male donations were directed for FFP production. The production of 100% male FFP was limited by the requirement to meet the national quality standard for FFP of 0.7 IU/mL of Factor VIII in >75% of units tested,[6] which can be met only by same-day processing. The proportion of male FFP has consistently been between 80% and 90% since implementation. Cryoprecipitate, containing only 30 to 50 mL of plasma per unit, continued to be made from female donors. As a variant Creutzfeldt-Jakob disease (vCJD) risk-reduction step, FFP for children began to be imported from the United States during 2004/2005. This plasma, which was all from male donors, was unpooled and virus inactivated using methylene blue. In 2006, a UK recommendation to use imported solvent/detergent-treated FFP (SDFFP) for plasma exchange procedures for TTP was issued to hospitals.

From 1996 until 2004, approximately 40% of adult platelet doses were provided from apheresis, with a gradual increase to 60% by the end of 2006. The remaining doses were produced from four pooled buffy coats, suspended in the plasma of one of the four donors. Beginning in October 2003, male plasma was preferentially used, contributing approximately 225 mL to each pool, with 25 mL each from the other three donors, who could be male or female. For manufacturing reasons, the use of male plasma for buffy-coat platelets was achieved in only 80% to 90% of pools. No specific steps were taken to reduce the risk from apheresis platelets.

As shown in Table 7-3, these component manufacturing changes have been associated with a gradual reduction in the total number of TRALI cases reported. The risk of highly likely or probable TRALI attributed to FFP associated with an antibody-positive donor fell dramatically, particularly after the "washout" period for female FFP still in storage. There were no concordant antibody-positive cases attributed to FFP in 2005 or 2006, although antibody-negative TRALI after FFP was occasionally reported. There was, however, a fatal antibody-positive case from cryoprecipitate in 2006. The reduction in the number of cases attributed to platelets was less dramatic, probably because no risk-reduction steps had been put in place for apheresis platelets. Four cases shown to be caused by antibody-positive female plasma in buffy-coat platelets occurred in 2004 and 2005, but none occurred in 2006.

As shown in Table 7-4, the risk of highly likely or probable TRALI associated with FFP and platelets has been reduced considerably since the preferentially male plasma policy was adopted, dropping from 15.5 to 3.2 per million components is-

Table 7-3. Changes to the Profile of TRALI Cases Reported to SHOT, 2003-2006

	2003	2004	2005	2006
TRALI Cases Analyzed	36	23	23	10
Highly likely	20	10	3	2
Probable	2	3	3	1
Possible	6	4	3	4
Unlikely	8	6	14	3
Implicated Component				
FFP	8	6	1	1
Platelets	8	4	2	1
Red cells	1	3	2	3
FFP + other	3	0	0	4
Cryo	1	0	1	1
Positive Donor Serology				
FFP	8	6	0	0
Platelets	8	3	3	1
Red cells	1	3	2	2
FFP + other	2	0	0	0
Cryo	1	0	1	1

SHOT = Serious Hazards of Transfusion (scheme); FFP = Fresh Frozen Plasma; cryo = cryoprecipitate.

sued for FFP/cryosupernatant (p = 0.0079) and from 14 to 5.8 per million components issued for platelets (p = 0.068). No such reduction was seen for red cells, where the male-to-female mix was unchanged, whereas for cryoprecipitate, the risk appears to have doubled. Although the numbers are small, this finding could be due to "enriching" of cryoprecipitate production with the female donors not used for FFP.

Table 7-4. Risk of Highly Likely and Probable Cases of TRALI before and after Introduction of Preferentially Male Plasma for FFP and Platelet Pools

	1999-2004	2004-2006
Red Cells Issued (000s)	13,411	4745
Cases implicating red cells	9	5
Cases/10^6 red cells issued (frequency)*	0.67 (1:1,490,000)	1.1 (1:949,000)[†]
FFP/Cryosupernatant Issued (000s)	1874	634
Cases implicating FFP/ cryosupernatant	29	2
Cases/10^6 FFP/cryosupernatant issued (frequency)*	15.5 (1:65,000)	3.2 (1:317,000)[‡]
Platelets Issued (000s)	1265	518
Cases implicating platelets	18	3
Cases/10^6 platelets issued (frequency)*	14 (1:71,000)	5.8 (1:173,000)[§]
Cryoprecipitate Issued (000s)	465	209
Cases implicating cryoprecipitate	2	2
Cases/10^6 cryoprecipitate issued (frequency)*	4.3 (1:232,000)	9.6 (1:104,000)[‖]

*Frequency calculated to nearest thousand.
[†]$p = 0.79$.
[‡]$p = 0.0079$.
[§]$p = 0.068$.
[‖]$p = 0.79$.
FFP = Fresh Frozen Plasma.

Discussion

There are limitations in using hemovigilance data to generate data on the incidence and causation of TRALI, but within these constraints the incidence of TRALI appears to be in the order of 1 case per 100,000 components. It is likely, however, that many cases are missed because of an underawareness on the part of clinicians. Conversely, in the absence of specific diagnostic criteria, observers with a particular interest in TRALI may overdiagnose the condition, which may lead to overreporting in the single hospital case series. The mortality in this series was 21% overall, which is at the high end of the 5% to 25% range in the reported series.[7] This may be because included were cases in which TRALI was thought to have been only a contributory factor to the death. The age range and diagnoses of the series cover the full range of patients likely to receive blood components. A previous nested case-control study has suggested an excess risk associated with cardiac surgery and hematologic malignancy.[8] On the basis of calculations from UK data on component usage (A Wells, EASTR study, unpublished observations), the authors' findings do not suggest a hugely increased risk in those groups of patients.

In 1999, SHOT introduced a likelihood scale that was based on both clinical features and serologic findings so that cases with positive donor or patient serology would fall into the probable or highly likely categories. The Canadian Consensus Conference proposed separate definitions for both TRALI and possible TRALI, but both are based entirely on clinical findings. Because there is scientific consensus that donor HLA or HNA antibodies are an important cause of TRALI, the authors believe that it is entirely legitimate to use serologic findings as part of the assessment of the likelihood of TRALI. This study's definitions resulted in approximately half the cases being classified as highly likely or probable.

By 2003, clear differences in risk emerged for different blood components, with the overall risk of TRALI from high plasma-volume components (FFP, cryosupernatant, and platelets) being 7 to 8 times higher than that for low plasma-volume components (red cells in additive solution and cryoprecipitate). When only highly likely or probable TRALI cases are considered, the excess risk from high plasma-volume components was 15 times higher. The authors did not see any differences in risk between pooled and apheresis platelets, probably because 75% of the plasma in pooled platelets comes from a single donor. Moreover, virtually all of the excess risk from FFP and platelets was associated with a serologically positive female donor. No cases were associated with previously transfused male donors. This may be related to the observation that HLA (and possibly HNA) antibodies induced by transfusion are of low affinity (mostly IgM) and tend to be transient when compared with those induced by pregnancy.[9] The strong association between female FFP, leukocyte antibodies, and TRALI was also noted in a recent series from the United States.[10] Furthermore, in the only prospective randomized trial in TRALI, plasma from parous females produced significantly greater reductions in oxygen saturation than control plasma, with one frank TRALI case.[11] However, although the implicated donor had granulocyte antibodies, a crossmatch with the patient specimen was negative.

Other important observations from the series are the findings of antibody-positive TRALI after red cell transfusion and of a fatality with transfusion of cryoprecipitate, confirming other evidence[10,12] that a small volume of antibody-positive plasma can cause TRALI. The cause of posttransfusion respiratory symptoms in antibody-negative cases remains unknown. Many cases had additional risk factors for ALI, and some may have had a degree of transfusion-associated circulatory overload (TACO). The SHOT assessment of suspected TRALI cases includes examination of fluid balance charts, but unless patients are in intensive care units, definitive diagnosis of TACO by measurement of pulmonary capillary wedge pressure is unlikely to be performed.

Some cases before 2001 could have been the result of HLA Class II antibodies; donors may have had HLA or HNA antibodies with titers below the limit of detection or have had other as-yet-undefined types of leukocyte antibodies. Finally, in cases associated with cellular blood components, there may have been accumulation of lipid-derived neutrophil-priming material during storage,[13,14] although the frequency with which the concentration of such material becomes capable of triggering a TRALI reaction remains undefined. Lipid-priming material has not been identified in FFP. TRALI caused by platelets has been reported to be associated with longer storage time, but this association was not investigated in the authors' series.[15]

Although the preferentially male plasma approach seems rather crude, it proved simple and of low cost to implement; this implementation was aided by certain characteristics of the UK blood supply. There was no program of FFP collection by apheresis, so male FFP could be implemented without loss of any donors. Because UK plasma cannot be used for fractionation as a result of vCJD risk, donors were already aware that most plasma was discarded, so the NBS did not specifically communicate the male plasma policy to donors. Similarly, suspending buffy-coat platelets in male plasma could be implemented relatively easily and again without a loss of donors. It has not yet proved possible to produce either 100% male FFP or plasma for platelet pools because of current UK requirements for production on the day of collection. Some other European countries have adopted the "20-C overnight hold of whole blood" method of component production, which produces red cells, platelets, and FFP of excellent quality.[16] Steps are being taken to introduce this method into the United Kingdom. An alternative strategy would be acceptance of "Day 1 FFP," as used in Canada.[17] The use of production strategies to reduce TRALI risk from FFP has been recommended by the AABB,[18] although not yet mandated by the Food and Drug Administration. This recommendation parallels the situation in Europe, where some blood services are moving voluntarily toward greater use of male FFP, without its being a European Union requirement.

The authors considered whether other factors may have contributed to the reduction in TRALI case reports to SHOT. Clinicians may have assumed that all FFP was male and therefore is no longer a TRALI risk, but the continued reporting of cases that can be tracked to a female donor does not suggest this. A further change was the recommended use of SDFFP for TTP.[19] Countries that have both heavy or universal use of SDFFP and an established hemovigilance system (Belgium, Ireland, Norway) have not reported any TRALI cases,[20] perhaps because of dilution of donations containing high-titer HLA or HNA antibodies, which are undetectable in the final product.[21] However, only about 10% of FFP is used for TTP (A Wells, EASTR study, unpublished observations), and uptake of SDFFP has not been complete, so the contribution of this policy is probably low. Appropriate prescribing of FFP and platelets is also being promoted. For example, UK guidelines for FFP recommend prothrombin complex concentrates for warfarin reversal in life-threatening situations, and vitamin K otherwise,[22] yet 5% of patients in this series developed TRALI after FFP was given to reverse warfarin. A systematic review of FFP trials concluded that no definite evidence for the benefit of FFP has been shown in high-quality trials in any clinical setting.[23] The relationship between abnormal coagulation, bleeding, and the role of FFP in preventing or treating hemorrhage remains uncertain,[24,25] and further studies are required to define it.

Finally, steps will be necessary to reduce TRALI resulting from transfusion of apheresis platelets. One possibility is the use of a platelet additive solution to replace most of the plasma. Several solutions are licensed in Europe, but none yet in the United States. Its effect in TRALI prevention, however, is uncertain because 100 mL of plasma are required in the final product. An alternative strategy would be to screen current apheresis donors for HLA and HNA antibodies, but this screening would result in loss of up to 7% to 10% of donors who have never caused TRALI. The United Kingdom has adopted an intermediate position by screening female prospective apheresis donors only. Perhaps a more refined approach would be to exclude donors with high-titer antibodies or those with specificities commonly associated with TRALI. No approach is ideal, but it is reassuring that, 15 years after risk reduction was recommended,[26] strategies are at last beginning to be discovered for overcoming one of the leading causes of transfusion-related mortality.

Summary

After seven years of evaluation of hemovigilance reports of TRALI in the United Kingdom, an association emerged between a TRALI episode and exposure to FFP or platelets from a female donor with HLA antibodies recognizing one or more recipient antigens. Consequently, in 2003/2004, a policy was introduced to produce FFP from male donors and to suspend platelet pools in male plasma as far as operationally possible (80% to 90% of components). This policy resulted in a fall in total TRALI reports, accounted for by the virtual elimination of TRALI caused by FFP and a reduction in cases caused by pooled platelets. There remains a need to reduce the risk of TRALI from apheresis platelets, either by HLA antibody screening or, perhaps, by the use of platelet additive solution.

Acknowledgments

The authors are grateful to all hospital staff who participate in SHOT and who reported TRALI cases; to the staff in UK histocompatibility and immunogenetics laboratories for performing the HLA and HNA investigations; to Dr. Cliff Morgan, Dr. Neil Soni, and Professor M. Mythen for clinical review of cases referred to SHOT; to Louise Choo for statistical support; to Neil Beckman for production data on use of male plasma; and to Rebecca Cardigan and the staff of the NBS Component Development Laboratory for calculations of plasma in platelet pools. Funding from the UK Blood Services is gratefully acknowledged.

References

1. Williamson LM, Heptonstall J, Soldan K. A SHOT in the arm for safer blood transfusion: A new surveillance system for transfusion hazards. Br Med J 1996;313:1221-2.
2. Kleinman S, Caulfield T, Chan P, et al. Toward an understanding of transfusion-related acute lung injury: Statement of a consensus panel. Transfusion 2004;44:1774-89.
3. Definitions of current SHOT categories and what to report. Manchester, UK: Serious Hazards of Transfusion scheme, 2008. [Available at http://www.shotuk.org/SHOT%20Categories%202008.pdf (accessed July 3, 2008).]
4. Lucas GF. Prospective evaluation of the chemiluminescence test for the detection of granulocyte antibodies: Comparison with the granulocyte immunofluorescence test. Vox Sang 1994;66:141-7.
5. MacLennan S, Lucas G, Brown C, et al. Prevalence of HLA and HNA antibodies in donors: Correlation with pregnancy and transfusion history. Vox Sang 2004;87(Suppl 3):S2-S16.
6. Statutory instrument 2005 no. 50: Blood safety and quality regulations 2005. Part 5: Quality and safety requirements for blood and blood components. Norwich, UK: Controller of Her Majesty's Stationery Office, 2005. Available at http://www.opsi.gov.uk/SI/si2005/20050050.htm (accessed July 2, 2008).]
7. Silliman CC, Ambruso DR, Boshkov LK. Transfusion-related acute lung injury. Blood 2005;105:2266-73.
8. Silliman CC, Boshkov LK, Mehdizadehkashi Z, et al. Transfusion-related acute lung injury: Epidemiology and a prospective analysis of etiologic factors. Blood 2003;101:454-62.
9. Brown C, Navarrete C. HLA antibody screening by LCT, LIFT and ELISA. In: Bidwell J, Navarrete C, eds. Histocompatibility testing. London: Imperial College Press, 2000:65-98.
10. Eder AF, Herron R, Strupp A, et al. Transfusion-related acute lung injury surveillance (2003-2005) and the potential impact of the selective use of plasma from male donors in the American Red Cross. Transfusion 2007:47:599-607.
11. Palfi M, Berg S, Ernerudh J, Berlin J. A randomized controlled trial of transfusion-related acute lung injury: Is plasma from multiparous blood donors dangerous? Transfusion 2001;41:317-22.
12. Win N, Ranasinghe E, Lucas G. Transfusion-related acute lung injury: A 5-year look-back study. Transfus Med 2002;12:387-9.
13. Silliman CC, Voelkel NF, Allard JD, et al. Plasma and lipids from stored packed red blood cells cause acute lung injury in an animal model. J Clin Invest 1998;101:1458-67.
14. Silliman CC, Bjornsen AJ, Wyman TH, et al. Plasma and lipids from stored platelets cause acute lung injury in an animal model. Transfusion 2003;43:633-40.
15. Andreu G, Morel P, Forestier F, et al. Hemovigilance network in France: Organization and analysis of immediate transfusion incident reports from 1994 to 1998. Transfusion 2002;42:1356-64.

16. Van der Meer PF, Pietersz RN. Overnight storage of whole blood: A comparison of two designs of butane-1,4-diol cooling plates. Transfusion 2007;47: 2038-43.

17. Cardigan R, Lawrie AS, Mackie IJ, Williamson LM. The quality of fresh-frozen plasma produced from whole blood stored at 4 degrees C overnight. Transfusion 2005;45:1342-8.

18. Transfusion-related acute lung injury. Association bulletin #06-07. Bethesda, MD: AABB, 2006. [Available at http://www.aabb.org/Content/Members_Area/Association_Bulletins/ab06-07.htm (accessed July 2, 2008).]

19. Allford SL, Hunt BJ, Rose P, Machin SJ. British Committee for Standards in Haematology: Guidelines on the diagnosis and management of the thrombotic microangiopathic haemolytic anaemias. Br J Haematol 2003;120:556-73.

20. Baudoux E, Margraff U, Coenen A, et al. Hemovigilance: Clinical tolerance of solvent-detergent treated plasma. Vox Sang 1998;74(Suppl 1):237-9.

21. Sachs UJ, Kauschat D, Bein G. White blood cell-reactive antibodies are undetectable in solvent/detergent plasma. Transfusion 2005;45:1628-31.

22. Guidelines for the use of fresh frozen plasma, cryoprecipitate and cryosupernatant. Br J Haematol 2004;126:11-28.

23. Stanworth SJ, Brunskill SJ, Hyde CJ, et al. Is Fresh Frozen Plasma clinically effective? A systematic review of randomized controlled trials. Br J Haematol 2004;126:139-52.

24. Segal JB, Dzik WH. Transfusion Medicine/Hemostasis Clinical Trials Network. Paucity of studies to support that abnormal coagulation test results predict bleeding in the setting of invasive procedures: An evidence-based review. Transfusion 2005;45:1413-25.

25. Abdel-Wahab OI, Healy B, Dzik WH. Effect of Fresh-Frozen Plasma transfusion on prothrombin time and bleeding in patients with mild coagulation abnormalities. Transfusion 2006;46:1279-85.

26. Popovsky MA, Chaplin HC Jr, Moore SB. Transfusion-related acute lung injury: A neglected, serious complication of hemotherapy. Transfusion 1992;32:589-92.

In: Kleinman S, Popovsky MA, eds.
TRALI: Mechanisms, Management, and Prevention
Bethesda, MD: AABB Press, 2008

8

TRALI Risk-Reduction Strategies

STEVEN KLEINMAN, MD, AND
DARRELL TRIULZI, MD

RECENT HEMOVIGILANCE DATA HAVE ESTAB-lished that transfusion-related acute lung injury (TRALI) is the number one cause of acute mortality from transfusion.[1-4] In the United States, reports of transfusion-related fatalities to the Food and Drug Administration (FDA) indicate that TRALI was the number one cause of fatalities in 2005 and 2006, with an average of 32 cases reported annually.[2] Previous estimates in the literature

Steven Kleinman, MD, Clinical Professor of Pathology, University of British Columbia School of Medicine, Vancouver, British Columbia, Canada, and Senior Medical Advisor, AABB, and Darrell Triulzi, MD, Medical Director, Institute for Transfusion Medicine, and Professor of Pathology, University of Pittsburgh School of Medicine, Pittsburgh, Pennsylvania suggest that annual mortality from TRALI may be much higher. Using a reported TRALI incidence of 1 in 5000 transfused components, a fatality rate of 5%, and 22 million components transfused annually in the United States, one can calculate that TRALI may be a contributing factor in 220 deaths annually.[5]

This situation is true in other countries as well. The 2005 UK Serious Hazards of Transfusion (SHOT) report lists TRALI as the leading cause of transfusion-related mortality, as does a recent report from the national Canadian Transfusion Transmitted Injuries Surveillance System (TTISS).[3,4]

The true incidence of TRALI is unknown. The most widely quoted figure is 1 in 5000 components. However, several recent reports from studies conducted in specific patient settings (eg, multiple intensive care units and in tertiary care hospitals) report an incidence of 1 in 1300 to 2400 transfused components if cases with other acute lung injury (ALI) risk factors are excluded, and 1 in 370 to 1000 transfused components if such cases are included.[6-9] A preliminary report from a prospective study being conducted at the University of California (UC)-San Francisco and the Mayo Clinic using an active surveillance method (prospective monitoring of patients who developed hypoxemia on the basis of computerized surveillance of blood gas measurements) found that TRALI incidence was approximately 1 in 3000 transfused components and 1 in 500 transfused patients.[6]

Preliminary Evidence for the Effectiveness of Enhanced TRALI Risk-Reduction Strategies

Several years ago, investigators from SHOT determined that the rate of TRALI occurrence in the United Kingdom was five- to sevenfold greater for blood components that contained high volumes of plasma [eg, Fresh Frozen Plasma (FFP) and buffy-coat-derived platelets resuspended in plasma from one of the donors in the pool] than for lower plasma-volume components [eg, additive solution Red Blood Cells (RBCs) and cryoprecipitate].[3,10] Their data also showed that most TRALI cases resulting from transfusion of the high plasma-volume components in-volved a leukocyte-antibody-positive female donor. On the basis of the SHOT analysis, the United Kingdom adopted a policy to minimize the transfusion of FFP and buffy-coat platelets from female donors. Since the implementation of this policy in Octo-ber 2003, the number of cases of TRALI arising from these components has decreased substantially. In 2003, there were 16 highly likely or probable cases where plasma or platelets were the implicated component; this number decreased to 10 cases in 2004 and 3 cases in 2005.[11]

The American Red Cross (ARC) analyzed 550 cases of sus-pected TRALI reported to that organization from 2003 through 2005.[12] All 72 reported fatalities were classified, without knowledge of the results of the associated serologic investiga-tion, by three physicians as either probable TRALI or of unre-lated etiology. A retrospective review of the fatal cases revealed 38 fatalities in which the diagnosis was probable TRALI; the majority (63%) occurred following plasma transfusion. A fe-male leukocyte-antibody-positive donor was involved in 75% (18 of 24) of cases involving plasma transfusion, in 60% of cases involving apheresis platelets (3 of 5), and in 71% (27 of 38) of all cases. Female antibody-positive donors were more likely to be associated with probable TRALI than with unre-lated cases [p = 0.0001; odds ratio (OR) = 9.5; 95% confi-dence interval (CI), 2.9-31.1]. The rate of probable TRALI among recipient fatalities was higher for plasma components (1:202,673; OR = 12.5; 95% CI, 5.4-28.9) and apheresis platelets (1:320,572; OR = 7.9; 95% CI, 2.5-24.8) compared to red cells (1:2,527,437). The analysis concluded that plasma transfusion was responsible for the majority of probable TRALI fatalities in the ARC system and that as many as 6 fatalities per year (or 47% of all TRALI fatalities) were linked to plasma from female donors with leukocyte antibodies.

Both of these sources of data indicated that the incidence of TRALI per unit transfused was higher for transfusable plasma components (eg, FFP) than for red cells. In the United Kingdom, the risk was also higher for buffy-coat platelets resuspended in the plasma of a single donor; in the United States, the risk was also higher for apheresis platelets. The data for whole-blood-derived platelets prepared by the platelet-rich plasma (PRP) method in the United States did not show an increased risk relative to red cells, but the numbers of such transfused components were limited. More recently, preliminary hemovigilance data from the Canadian TTISS reported that the incidence of TRALI from pooled whole-blood-derived PRP platelets, when expressed per platelet transfusion dose (eg, a pool of 5 platelet concentrates), was similar to that for apheresis platelets.[4]

In addition to the data from passive reporting systems, at least two recent studies (one retrospective and one prospective) conducted in the intensive care unit (ICU) setting concluded that patients with TRALI and possible TRALI received a greater total volume of plasma as well as a higher volume of plasma from female donors than did control patients.[7,8] After logistic regression modeling, these donor factors were predictive of risk for the development of TRALI or possible TRALI in each of these studies. In addition, the number of pregnancies in donors whose plasma was transfused was also predictive in the prospective study. These studies support the results of the one small randomized control trial that evaluated the adverse clinical events associated with transfusion of plasma from multiparous females vs plasma from never pregnant females in 105 ICU patients. This study showed an increased incidence of transfusion reactions (including one case of TRALI) as well as a small but statistically significant decrease in partial pressure of oxygen in arterial blood/inspired oxygen concentration (PaO_2/FiO_2) following transfusion of plasma from multiparous donors when compared to transfusion of control plasma.[13]

Policy Evolution

International Developments

As early as 1992, some authors raised the issue that TRALI was a serious enough problem to warrant changes in blood component production by minimizing the number of transfusable plasma components that were collected from multiparous females.[14,15] However, with rare exceptions (eg, single institutions in Spain and the Netherlands), this policy was not implemented.[16,17] Instead, until recently, TRALI risk-reduction strategies throughout the world depended on minimizing non-indicated transfusions and deferring donors who were found to be implicated as the presumed causative donor in a TRALI case. A donor was defined as implicated if a serologic workup demonstrated an HLA or human neutrophil antigen (HNA) antibody in the donor and a corresponding cognate antigen in the recipient, or if a leukocyte crossmatch was positive.[18]

There appear to be at least three reasons that more extensive TRALI risk-reduction strategies have been implemented recently in many countries. First, TRALI now clearly stands as the statistically highest severe transfusion risk, which was not the case in the 1990s. Second, the UK experience has suggested that the preferential male plasma approach is efficacious. Third, over the past decade, the transfusion medicine community has implemented logistically complicated and very expensive interventions [minipool nucleic acid testing (NAT) for human immunodeficiency virus (HIV) and hepatitis C virus (HCV) and automated bacterial culturing of apheresis and buffy-coat platelets] to further reduce other risks that were as low as, or lower than, the current TRALI risk. Therefore, the operational complexity of a TRALI risk-reduction program does not seem as daunting as it may have been more than a decade ago.[19]

The major aim of recently proposed TRALI risk-reduction strategies is to lower TRALI risk without compromising the availability of needed blood components. Because component availability varies between jurisdictions, there is no universally applicable specific TRALI risk reduction strategy for all blood collection facilities. In some jurisdictions, an incremental approach to TRALI risk-reduction may be necessary in order to guarantee an adequate supply of a particular blood component.

In October 2003, the United Kingdom initiated its policy of providing preferentially male-donor transfusable plasma and buffy-coat platelet components. In 2004, before having any evaluable data from the UK experience, the Canadian TRALI Consensus Conference Panel was asked to address the question of TRALI risk-reduction policies.[20] The panel did not recommend that action should be taken but did recommend that blood collection facilities should evaluate whether interventions to reduce TRALI risk (eg, using male plasma rather than female plasma for transfusion, excluding plasma from multiparous females from transfusion, or excluding plasma from donors with HLA antibodies) would have a projected benefit that would be in excess of any potential adverse impact, such as a decrease in the availability of needed blood components.

AABB Recommendations

By the fall of 2006, data from the United Kingdom had demonstrated a reduction in TRALI cases associated with diversion of female plasma, and ARC data suggested that the majority of the fatal TRALI cases reported to ARC were associated with female plasma donors.[11,12] Prompted by these data, in November 2006, the AABB issued a set of recommendations for TRALI risk reduction for recipients of high plasma-volume components.[21] The specific recommendations were listed in an *Association Bulletin* as follows[21]:

1. Blood collecting facilities should implement interventions to minimize the preparation of high plasma-volume components from donors known to be leukocyte-alloimmunized or at increased risk of leukocyte alloimmunization.
2. Blood collection facilities should work toward implementing appropriate evidence-based hemotherapy practices in order to minimize unnecessary transfusion.
3. Blood collection and transfusion facilities should monitor the incidence of reported TRALI and TRALI-related mortality.

The *Bulletin* clearly stated that, on the basis of the current state of knowledge, no set of available interventions could eliminate TRALI. It is now widely accepted that there are at least two different and incompletely understood pathophysiologic mechanisms (leukocyte antibody-mediated and nonantibody-mediated) that can cause TRALI.[22] The first AABB recommendation concerning component manufacturing risk-reduction strategies targeted these strategies toward antibody-mediated TRALI. This course of action was based on an interpretation of the available clinical data, which suggested that the antibody-mediated mechanism is the most common mechanism of TRALI and that antibody-mediated TRALI is clinically more severe and more often leads to mortality than does TRALI caused by the nonantibody mechanism. Furthermore, there were no data to support any specific interventions for preventing nonantibody-mediated TRALI, other than to decrease nonindicated transfusions.[23,24]

The first of the three AABB recommendations was directed toward all transfusable high plasma-volume components [FFP; Plasma Frozen Within 24 Hours After Phlebotomy (FP-24); and Plasma, Cryoprecipitate Reduced] as well as platelet components that contain high volumes of plasma from a single donor—specifically, Apheresis Platelets and buffy-coat-derived platelets resuspended in plasma. The extension of the recommendation to these platelet components was based on data (reported earlier) from the United Kingdom and the United States as well as the observation that FFP, buffy-coat-derived platelets, and Apheresis Platelets all contain a minimum of 200 mL of plasma. For a similar reason, the recommendation was also applied to whole blood, which is infrequently transfused. There were few data to permit the evaluation of TRALI risk posed by platelet concentrates prepared by the PRP method. In the United States, each such unit contains between 50 and 70 mL of plasma from a single donor; these are usually administered to a recipient in pools of 4 to 6 units. The ARC data assessing fatal cases of TRALI found the per-unit risk for an individual platelet concentrate (rather than a platelet pool) to be equivalent to that of an RBC unit.[12] Thus, the recommendation to minimize transfusions from donors known to be leukocyte-alloimmunized or at increased risk of leukocyte alloimmunization was not extended to donors of PRP platelets.

The ARC and UK data sets showed a much lower per-unit risk for red cells and for cryoprecipitate than for plasma; thus, no specific manufacturing interventions were recommended for these components. However, because of the number of RBC units transfused, it has been well documented that this component appears responsible for the largest number of TRALI cases.[4] Clearly, preventing TRALI from red cell transfusion is a highly desirable goal; however, there is no practical intervention that can be applied to modify this risk. Interventions such as using predominantly male donors or screening selected donors for HLA antibodies would severely compromise red cell availability.

Results of Policy Implementation

A recently published survey of experts from 14 countries addressed planned TRALI risk-reduction policies as of late 2006.[25] Most respondents (primarily from European countries) indicated that they were planning either to reduce the percentage of transfused plasma units from female donors or to completely eliminate such transfusions. Several European respondents indicated that they currently use or plan to use solvent/detergent-treated (SD) plasma. Most respondents did not indicate plans to implement similar TRALI risk-reduction policies for apheresis platelets.

A September 2007 survey administered to AABB member institutions in the United States found that most institutions had partially or fully implemented a TRALI risk-reduction strategy for transfusable plasma components [ie, predominantly male or exclusively male plasma (see below)] but that only a few institutions had as yet implemented a TRALI risk-reduction strategy for apheresis platelets.[26]

Risk Reduction by Improving Transfusion Practice

Transfusion medicine specialists have repeatedly stressed that the decision to transfuse should be based on a risk/benefit analysis for an individual patient as well as on the principles of evidence-based medicine. In recent years, several sets of transfusion guidelines that were based on a critical review of the literature have been developed by expert groups. Knowledge and application of these current transfusion guidelines by transfusing physicians will serve to maximize the benefit of transfusion while minimizing the needless exposure of patients to the risks of transfusion, including TRALI. To the extent possible, transfusion medicine physicians should attempt to influence clinicians to transfuse blood components appropriately.

Guidelines for prophylactic platelet transfusion in hematology-oncology patients have been well established on the basis of multiple randomized controlled trials (RCTs) showing that stable patients can be safely supported using a prophylactic transfusion trigger of 10,000/µL.[27-30] Patients with complicating factors that consume platelets or shorten platelet survival (such as high fever, sepsis, disseminated intravascular coagulation, splenomegaly, or bleeding) warrant transfusion at a higher threshold, typically 20,000/µL. For bleeding patients with thrombocytopenia, observational studies have shown that hemostasis was effectively achieved when platelet transfusions raised the platelet count above 50,000/µL.[31,32] The threshold for platelet transfusion in other patient populations with bleeding or undergoing invasive procedures has not been as well established. Retrospective studies suggest that patients can safely undergo minor surgical procedures such as paracentesis, thoracentesis, or liver biopsy with platelet counts above 50,000/µL.[33,34] In a retrospective observational study of 167 surgical procedures in patients with acute leukemia and thrombocytopenia, Bishop et al observed no excess surgical bleeding for patients with platelet counts >50,000/µL.[35] Thus, although 50,000/µL is typically recommended for patients with bleeding or planned surgery, this guideline is not supported by any RCT in the nonhematology-oncology population undergoing surgery.[36,37]

Guidelines for plasma transfusion are also largely based on observational studies and a paucity of RCTs.[38,39] Published guidelines typically recommend plasma transfusion therapy for patients who are bleeding or undergoing an invasive procedure and have a prothrombin time (PT) greater than 1.5 times the midpoint of the normal range, translating approximately to an international normalized ratio (INR) >1.6.[36] Plasma therapy is typically used to treat coagulopathy in one of two clinical scenarios: bleeding or a planned invasive procedure. The assumptions underlying current practice are that abnormalities of the PT/INR correlate with the risk of bleeding and that plasma therapy can correct the abnormal PT/INR, thereby reducing or eliminating the risk of bleeding. A review of the literature by Segal and Dzik yielded 24 observational studies and one clinical trial examining PT/INR and bleeding.[38] They concluded that the data did not support the utility of PT/INR in predicting bleeding. Stanworth et al provided a literature review of RCTs examining the clinical effectiveness of plasma therapy for procedure prophylaxis or bleeding.[39] Only 17 trials compared FFP to no FFP or a colloid solution in adults; 10 of these studies were in cardiac surgery. No study demonstrated a significant difference in either laboratory or clinical outcomes in those receiving plasma. Therefore, although published guidelines recommend plasma therapy for patients with an INR of 1.5 to 2.0, the literature lacks RCT data to support this practice. A renewed emphasis on monitoring plasma transfusion practice should be an important component of a TRALI risk-reduction strategy.

In the absence of specific recommended interventions to reduce the incidence of TRALI from red cell transfusions, appropriate use with the avoidance of nonindicated transfusions remains the best course of action. In contrast to decision-making for platelet and plasma transfusion, routinely available laboratory data (eg, hemoglobin/hematocrit) are of less value in making the decision to transfuse red cells. Thus, red cell transfusion decisions are based more on clinical judgment, as noted in published guidelines.[40-42] Three recent well-designed prospective RCTs have helped define the optimal transfusion threshold in terms of mortality in adult ICU, pediatric ICU, and postoperative cardiac surgery patients.[43-45] All three studies suggest that these patients do not benefit from transfusions at hemoglobin >9.0 g/dL and should not be transfused until hemoglobin values are in the 7 to 8 g/dL range. These studies did not include patients with acute coronary syndromes (including acute myocardial infarction), and the transfusion threshold in such patients remains controversial.[46,47] No prospective RCTs address more subtle potential benefits from transfusion, such as improved physical status or recovery from surgery. Thus, the optimal transfusion thresholds for patients such as those with chronic obstructive pulmonary disease, those with congestive heart failure, or those recovering from orthopedic surgery are not clear. A National Institutes of Health (NIH)-funded multicenter study of red cell transfusion in orthopedic surgery patients with a history of coronary artery disease is under way.[48]

Risk Reduction for Plasma Components

Plasma Manufactured from Whole Blood

Plasma for transfusion is supplied either as a component manufactured from a whole blood collection or a component collected by apheresis. Plasma is either frozen within 8 hours (as FFP) or Frozen Within 24 Hours After Phlebotomy (FP-24) to preserve coagulation factor activity. Multiple studies have shown that FFP and FP-24 are essentially equivalent components for the treatment of almost all conditions requiring coagulation factor replacement.[49]

With regard to transfusable plasma components manufactured from whole blood, the primary strategy for reducing TRALI risk has been to transfuse units that were manufactured exclusively or predominantly from male donors. This strategy is viable because of the excess of plasma products produced from whole blood; after processing, male plasma can be targeted for transfusion, whereas female plasma can be shipped as recovered plasma and used for further manufacture into plasma derivatives. In the United States, for the common blood groups (groups A and O), this strategy appears to be readily accomplishable without creating any shortages of transfusable plasma components. In some blood centers that collect blood over large geographic areas that are some distance from the component production laboratory, the logistics of targeting male plasma for transfusion are made easier if FP-24 is supplied rather than FFP.[49]

The approach of targeting male plasma for transfusion does not require any additional questioning of donors but merely requires that a mechanism exists to distinguish male from female units as they pass through the component production laboratory. Because the final plasma component is not labeled as coming from a male or female donor and because no absolute safety claim is made, plasma from female donors can also be released for transfusion if logistic considerations make this necessary. This release is more likely to occur with group AB and, to a lesser extent, group B plasma, as these components are more likely to be in short supply. To avoid component shortages, some blood centers may adopt a strategy of transfusing plasma from females who have never been pregnant, as well as from males, because such female donors would also have a very low risk of having been alloimmunized and of developing leukocyte antibodies. This latter strategy necessitates obtaining a pregnancy history from female donors, which involves adding a question to the donor history questionnaire.

Implementation of the predominantly male plasma strategy has not required any special communication with individual whole blood donors because the red cells from donations by both male and female donors are still used for transfusion, and the plasma is used either for transfusion or for further manufacture.

Plasma Collected by Apheresis

Transfusable plasma components can also be obtained from a dedicated plasmapheresis procedure or from a combined apheresis procedure (involving the collection of multiple components). On the basis of FDA rules, blood collection facilities without a source plasma license can use such plasma only for transfusion. Therefore, a TRALI risk-reduction strategy for this component involves a decision about whether to collect plasma from the donor. Plasmapheresis programs have thus 1) eliminated the use of female donors, 2) restricted collections to female donors without a history of pregnancy, or 3) determined that component availability considerations (ie, for group AB plasma) require that some plasma be collected from previously pregnant female donors. In the latter case, such previously pregnant donors may in the future be subject to the same type of HLA antibody testing that is likely to be performed for apheresis platelet donors (see below).

Solvent/Detergent-Treated Plasma

An alternate strategy for reducing TRALI risk from transfused plasma is to use pooled SD plasma in place of single-donor plasma. The data establishing the safety profile of this component with regard to TRALI have been accumulating over the past several years. First, reports from countries that transfuse SD plasma have indicated an absence of TRALI from SD plasma, despite the transfusion of several million units. However, these reports are either anecdotal, are referenced as being on file with the component manufacturer, or have been presented at symposia funded by the manufacturer of the component.[50,51] Such reports have not yet appeared in the peer-reviewed medical literature. More recently, data from the French hemovigilance system also support the contention that SD plasma does not carry a risk for TRALI. Both single-donor FFP and SD plasma are transfused in France. In the past 4 years, using standardized and uniform criteria, the French hemovigilance system has documented TRALI following FFP infusion but not following the infusion of over 400,000 doses of SD plasma (G Andreu, personal communication).[52] Two in-vitro studies of one manufacturer's SD plasma product (OctaPlas, OctaPharma, Lachen, Switzerland) have shown that no HLA antibody was detectable in 32 screened batches.[51,53] This may be the result of dilution of the HLA antibody present in some plasma units by virtue of pooling with 500 to 1600 other plasma units or the binding of HLA antibody to soluble HLA antigen present in plasma from other donor units in the pool, or both.

The decision to transfuse SD plasma depends on many additional factors unrelated to TRALI risk reduction. European formulations of SD plasma have much higher levels of protein S activity compared to previously approved US formulations. These low US levels may have led to an increased risk of thrombosis associated with the US product.[54] Currently, an FDA-licensed SD plasma product is not available in the United States.

Risk Reduction for Platelet Components

Apheresis Platelets

TRALI risk-reduction approaches for apheresis platelets will need to balance reducing TRALI risk against ensuring adequate availability of platelets for transfusion. This is a significant issue in the United States, where 80% of platelet transfusions are with apheresis platelets; this number is rising to 100% in some regions of the country.[55] Most US blood collection centers have an insufficient number of male plateletpheresis donors to fully support apheresis platelet collections. This will be true even as attempts are made to recruit more male plateletpheresis donors, to more frequently collect apheresis platelets from these donors, and to make a greater number of split apheresis components from these collections. Therefore, some female plateletpheresis donors will continue to be needed, and a TRALI risk-reduction strategy will almost certainly need to include a procedure to identify and continue to collect platelets from female donors who have a low likelihood of alloimmunization to leukocyte antigens. As part of this strategy, current female apheresis donors who have a high likelihood of alloimmunization or who have been demonstrated to be alloimmunized by detection of HLA antibodies would be diverted from apheresis donation to whole blood donation. This same strategy could also be applied to screening current female plasmapheresis donors, either in general or for specific blood groups such as group AB.

The November 2006 AABB recommendations suggested that possible approaches to achieving TRALI risk reduction for plateletpheresis donors could involve questioning donors about pregnancy history, testing donors for HLA antibody, or a combination of these approaches (ie, using pregnancy history to triage donors for HLA antibody testing).[21] This latter suggestion was based on several studies showing that the frequency of HLA antibodies increases with the number of pregnancies.[56,57] The *Association Bulletin* indicated that very little data existed to evaluate whether a history of transfusion in a donor (ie, transfusion at least 12 months before donation) was a significant risk factor for the presence of HLA antibody.

Platelets and HLA Antibody Testing

Who Should Be Tested?

A potential strategy to minimize TRALI from apheresis donors is to obtain a history of potentially alloimmunizing events (eg, pregnancy or transfusion) and test donors with alloimmunization risk factors for leukocyte antibodies. Previous studies of the prevalence of HLA antibodies in blood donors with a history of pregnancy or transfusion used test methods that are less sensitive than current assays or were hampered by insufficient sample sizes.[56,57] The Leukocyte Antibody Prevalence Study (LAPS) has recently been conducted by the National Heart, Lung, and Blood Institute's Retrovirus Epidemiology Donor Study-II (REDS-II) network to measure the prevalence of HLA antibodies in blood donors with or without a history of blood transfusion or pregnancy, using sensitive flow cytometry methods.[58] Donors completed a self-administered survey of their transfusion history and their detailed pregnancy history, including early terminations, miscarriages, or tubal pregnancies. Each donor provided a sample of blood to be tested for the presence and specificity of HLA Class I and Class II antibodies using a flow cytometry platform (Luminex, Luminex Corp, Austin, TX) and silicon beads coated with cell-culture-derived HLA antigens (One Lambda, Canoga Park, CA). Over a 6-month period from December 2006 to May 2007, a total of 8171 whole blood and apheresis donors were enrolled in the study (D Triulzi, unpublished observations).[59] There were 7920 valid samples for HLA antibody analysis.

The study found that transfusion had only a minimal effect on Class I or Class II HLA antibody prevalence as assessed by comparing results in males with and without a history of having received a blood transfusion. The prevalence of any HLA antibody (Class I, Class II, or both) was low in both the transfused and nontransfused groups (1.7% vs 1.0%). The effect of pregnancy on the rate of HLA alloimmunization is shown in Fig 8-1. There is a clear and significant increase in the prevalence of HLA Class I, Class II, or any HLA antibody from zero to four or more pregnancies (p <0.0001). Women who reported never being pregnant or transfused had a low rate of HLA antibody alloimmunization (1.7%), which was similar to the rate for male donors (D Triulzi, unpublished observations).

These data indicate that—for the purpose of identifying donors at increased risk of HLA alloimmunization—transfused males and never-pregnant females are similar to nontransfused males. Thus, there appears to be no significantly increased value in adopting a TRALI risk-reduction strategy that involves HLA antibody testing of donors who have not had at least one previous pregnancy. Restricting HLA antibody testing using Luminex to female apheresis donors with a history of previous pregnancy is predicted to result in a loss of approximately 16.2% of female apheresis donors (D Triulzi, unpublished observations). Ongoing analyses will determine whether the type of pregnancy and the time since the last pregnancy affect alloimmunization rates.

Other Issues

In addition to determining who should be tested, other issues with regard to HLA antibody testing include which test method

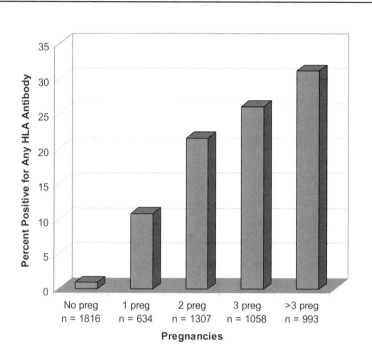

Figure 8-1. Effect of pregnancy on the rate of HLA antibody prevalence in female blood donors enrolled in the Leukocyte Antibody Prevalence Study. HLA Class I and Class II antibody testing was performed on plasma samples using One Lambda LabScreen Mixed reagents on a Luminex platform. A result was interpreted as positive if one or more beads coated with antigens for a given HLA class (Class I or Class II) gave a value for the normalized background ratio (NBG) that was greater than the mean plus 3 standard deviations of the natural log transformed distribution of NBG values in the 1138 nontransfused male blood donors tested as part of this study. Based on this analysis, samples with an NBG >10.8 for any Class I multi-antigen bead were considered positive for HLA Class I antibody, and those with an NBG >6.9 for any Class II multi-antigen bead were considered positive for HLA Class II antibody. The percentages of donors with any antibody (HLA Class I, II, or both) were compared for female donors with different numbers of pregnancies (1816 donors with zero pregnancies, 634 donors with one pregnancy, 1307 donors with two pregnancies, 1058 donors with three pregnancies, and 993 donors with four or more pregnancies). The results were statistically significant (p <0.0001) for the relationship between HLA antibody prevalence and the increasing number of pregnancies.

should be used, how often such testing should be conducted, whether donors should be notified of their results, and whether HLA antibody-positive donors should be diverted to whole blood donation.

HLA antibody detection has historically been performed using the lymphocytotoxicity assay (LCA), usually with antiglobulin enhancement.[60] More recently, the detection of HLA Class I or Class II antibodies in TRALI has involved a solid phase assay, an HLA enzyme-linked immunosorbent assay,[61] or the flow panel reactive assay.[62] LCA is less sensitive than the other methods and may miss noncytotoxic HLA antibodies.[63] The flow-based microbead assay uses purified Class I or Class II HLA antigen-coated microbeads. Antigen-specific beads can be used to determine antibody specificity. This method has been adapted for high throughput and has been recommended by some as the standard for HLA antibody testing for donor investigations in TRALI case workups.[63]

The persistence of HLA antibodies is of interest in determining how often testing should be performed. The limited available data suggest that donors who are positive for HLA antibodies will remain positive. A small pilot study of multiparous females with strong HLA antibodies found persistence of antibody for more than 10 years.[64] The LAPS will provide additional data regarding the effect of the time since the last immunizing event on the prevalence of HLA antibodies. The preliminary results suggest that donors who have a negative test result for HLA antibodies could reasonably be tested again only if they report a pregnancy since their last test.

Because approximately 15% of previously pregnant apheresis donors will have HLA antibodies, a management strategy for these donors is needed.[59] It appears likely that the favored strategy will be to divert these donors to donation of whole blood, with the production of RBCs from such donations for transfusion. These whole blood donations should not be used for producing transfusable plasma components. There is not yet a consensus regarding the production of whole blood platelets from these "diverted" donors. In favor of using such platelets are the following facts: whole blood donations by previously pregnant donors are currently used for platelet production, there are no plans to screen previously pregnant whole blood donors for HLA antibody, and data from the ARC suggest that whole-blood-derived platelets are a low risk component.[12] Reasons to exclude diverted donors from platelet production include the following: the preliminary Canadian data suggest that there may be a higher TRALI risk from pooled platelets than previously thought,[4] and the numbers of whole-blood-derived platelets lost from "diverted" donors would have minimal effects on platelet supply. In the absence of any specific recommendations to the contrary, production of whole-blood-derived platelets from diverted donors is likely to continue.[26]

A policy regarding donor notification should be developed for donors discovered to have HLA antibodies. If such donors will no longer be eligible to donate apheresis platelets or plasma, they should be notified concerning why they are ineligible and should be educated about the significance of TRALI. The implications of having HLA antibodies on donor health are not significant and are not likely to affect many donors. Such donors may be at increased risk for stem cell or organ rejection should they need a transplant. They may also be at increased risk for febrile reactions, should they need a transfusion, and possibly for the development of TRALI from granulocyte transfusions. LAPS data show that 15% of previously pregnant women have detectable HLA antibodies, and no current clinical standard of care recommends notification of these women in other settings in which HLA antibody is detected. Thus, the most compelling reason for notification is to alert the donor to a change in donation status.

Platelets and HNA Antibody Testing

HNA antibodies, particularly anti-HNA-3a (formerly designated as granulocyte 5b), have been implicated in a number of TRALI cases.[22] Testing for neutrophil-specific antibodies is problematic in that the most commonly used methods are labor-intensive manual assays that require fresh human granulocytes, and there is inadequate standardization of methodology and interpretation.[60,65] Assays that are being used include granulocyte agglutination, granulocyte immunofluorescence by manual or flow cytometry techniques, and monoclonal antibody immobilization of neutrophil antigens (MAINA).[60] Testing is complicated by the fact that HLA antibodies may interfere with current methods and may require adsorption with platelets. Flow cytometry using cloned antigens is promising, but the 3a antigen has yet to be cloned. Prior studies of the prevalence of neutrophil-specific antibodies in previously pregnant donors have reported a low prevalence, which ranges between 0.1% and 1.8%.[57,66] These data suggest that the logistics of testing with current methods for such a low antibody prevalence will not be practical. The LAPS will be assessing the prevalence of HNA antibodies in a subset of donors who have no history of an alloimmunizing event and in multiparous female donors with and without HLA antibodies. It is expected that the LAPS data will provide a basis for determining whether HNA testing is likely to be useful.

Buffy-Coat-Derived Platelets

Buffy-coat platelets are routinely resuspended in the plasma from one of the donors included in the pooled component, usually derived from four or five donors. Thus, risk reduction for this component can be achieved by using plasma from a male donor (rather than a female donor) to resuspend the pool, which is the approach that has been adopted in the United Kingdom. The contribution of plasma from the other platelet concentrates in the pool is minimal, effectively making these low plasma-volume components.

Platelet-Additive Solutions

One other potential strategy to reduce TRALI risk from apheresis or buffy-coat platelets is to store these components in platelet-additive storage solutions, which reduce plasma volume by approximately two-thirds. As yet, no data exist to evaluate whether reduction of this amount of plasma volume will have an effect on the incidence of antibody-mediated TRALI.[67] Currently, several platelet-additive storage solutions are in use in Europe, but none are licensed in the United States.

Other Possible Measures for TRALI Prevention

The measures discussed earlier focus on the risk of TRALI related to leukocyte antibodies in blood donors. Leukocyte antibodies have been implicated in the large majority of, but not all, cases of TRALI. In addition, TRALI may be caused by the "two-hit" mechanism, which posits that transfusion of blood components containing biologic response modifiers (BRMs) capable of priming and/or activating neutrophils and possibly the endothelium can induce TRALI in a susceptible recipient.[22,68] BRMs implicated in clinical cases or animal models of TRALI include lysophosphatidyl choline (LPC), bacterial-derived lipopolysaccharides, cytokines, chemokines, growth factors, CD40-ligand, immune complexes, and leukocyte antibodies. The complex interplay between these molecules and recipient neutrophils and endothelium is incompletely understood; however, the proposed two-hit mechanism has led to consideration of other potential interventions to prevent TRALI.

Leukocyte Reduction

Popovsky and Moore[5] reported that 6% of cases were associated with *recipient* leukocyte antibodies directed at transfused neutrophils. This phenomenon has only rarely been reported since then and has been associated primarily with granulocyte transfusions.[68,69] Leukocyte reduction does not affect the accumulation of implicated BRMs such as LPC and CD40-ligand. Additional data are needed to assess whether leukocyte reduction affects the accumulation of other potential BRMs. Therefore, available data do not support routine leukocyte reduction as a method to reduce the risk of TRALI.

Use of Fresh Components

Because of the accumulation of BRMs during storage of red cells and platelets, transfusion of fresh components in susceptible recipients has been suggested.[24] This approach has not been widely adopted because of the incomplete understanding of patient risk factors, of the effect of duration of storage and component preparation on BRMs, and of the interplay between infused BRMs, host factors, and clinical TRALI.

Washed Blood Components

Washing would remove BRMs, including leukocyte antibodies, from cellular blood components. This approach has significant logistic and cost implications that include loss of cell mass (ie, for either platelets or red cells) and, in the case of platelets, possible loss of component quality. For these reasons, routine washing cannot be recommended at this time. However, cell washing may be used in selected recipients felt to be at high risk for TRALI on the basis of clinical judgment.

Monitoring the Effects of Interventions

Careful monitoring of TRALI incidence is necessary to obtain data for an assessment of the effectiveness of TRALI risk-reduction interventions. The importance of this approach has been illustrated by conclusions that have been drawn from the SHOT data.

To facilitate the collection of meaningful data, institutions should standardize their investigations of suspected TRALI cases. Physicians must be familiar with standardized clinical definitions of TRALI and its differentiation from transfusion-associated circulatory overload. High-quality reporting systems are necessary on the hospital level in order to capture clinical cases of suspected TRALI, and detailed reporting from the hospital to the blood center is also needed so that donor evaluations can be conducted and regional case data can be tabulated. Monitoring the effectiveness of TRALI interventions on a national basis will depend on the robustness of the national hemovigilance system that is in place. It should be noted that trends in TRALI incidence data may be difficult to interpret because the incidence may appear to increase as a result of enhanced case recognition, reporting, or both, thereby masking an actual decreased incidence because of risk-reduction strategies. However, this confounding effect was not seen in the United Kingdom, where the national hemovigilance system had focused on TRALI for 5 years before implementation of the UK risk-reduction strategy.[3]

Summary

TRALI is the leading cause of transfusion-related mortality. Recent studies also suggest that the incidence of nonfatal TRALI may be higher than previously documented, especially in seriously ill patient populations. These observations have resulted in focused attention from the transfusion medicine community on TRALI risk reduction. In addition to emphasis on the need for transfusions to be given only when indicated, recent risk-reduction policies include strategies to collect and/or manufacture particular blood components from donors with a probable decreased risk of causing TRALI. Preliminary experience from the United Kingdom has strongly suggested that restricting the manufacture of transfusable plasma components (eg, FFP) from female donors has reduced TRALI incidence. This observation has led to widespread international implementation of a similar TRALI risk-reduction strategy (ie, all-male plasma, predominantly male plasma, or SD plasma) in many countries. Reducing the risk of TRALI from transfusion of apheresis platelets is more problematic because the availability of this blood component would be severely affected by a strategy that restricted collection to male donors only. In the United States, consideration is being given to screening some (based on previous pregnancy history) or all female plateletpheresis donors for HLA antibody and to diverting those with antibody to whole blood donation. The effect of these new interventions on TRALI incidence is currently unknown and will be determined only if careful data-gathering efforts can be conducted over the next several years.

References

1. Holness L, Knippen MA, Simmons L, Lachenbruch PA. Fatalities caused by TRALI. Transfus Med Rev 2004;18:184-8.
2. Food and Drug Administration. Fatalities reported to the FDA following blood collection and transfusion: Annual summary for fiscal years 2005 and 2006. Rockville, MD: Center for Biologics Evaluation and Research, 2008. [Available at http://www.fda.gov/cber/blood/fatal0506.htm (accessed July 7, 2008).]
3. Stainsby D, Jones H, Asher D, et al. Serious hazards of transfusion: A decade of hemovigilance in the UK. Transfus Med Rev 2006;20:273-82.
4. Robillard P, McCombie N. TRALI, possible TRALI, and respiratory complications of transfusion reported to the Canadian Transfusion Transmitted Injuries Surveillance System (abstract). Transfusion 2007;47(Suppl 3S):5A.
5. Popovsky MA, Moore SB. Diagnostic and pathogenetic considerations in transfusion-related acute lung injury. Transfusion 1985;25:573-7.
6. Toy P, Gajic O, Gropper M, et al. Prospective assessment of the incidence of TRALI (abstract). Transfusion 2007;47(Suppl 3S):7A.
7. Rana R, Fernandez-Perez ER, Khan SA, et al. Transfusion-related acute lung injury and pulmonary edema in critically ill patients: A retrospective study. Transfusion 2006;46:1478-83.
8. Gajic O, Rana R, Winters JL, et al. Transfusion-related acute lung injury in the critically ill: Prospective nested case-control study. Am J Respir Crit Care Med 2007;176:886-91.
9. Finlay HE, Cassorla L, Feiner J, Toy P. Designing and testing a computer-based screening system for transfusion-related acute lung injury. Am J Clin Pathol 2005;124:601-9.
10. Goldman M, Webert KE, Arnold DM, et al. Proceedings of a consensus conference: Towards an understanding of TRALI. Transfus Med Rev 2005;19:2-31.

11. Chapman CE, Williamson LM, Cohen H, et al. The impact of using male donor plasma on hemovigilance reports of transfusion related acute lung injury (TRALI) in the UK (abstract). Vox Sang 2006;91(Suppl 3):227.

12. Eder AF, Herron R, Strupp A, et al. Transfusion-related acute lung injury surveillance (2003-2005) and the potential impact of the selective use of plasma from male donors in the American Red Cross. Transfusion 2007;47:599-607.

13. Palfi M, Berg S, Ernerudh J, Berlin G. A randomized controlled trial of transfusion-related acute lung injury: Is plasma from multiparous blood donors dangerous? Transfusion 2001;41:317-22.

14. Popovsky MA, Chaplin HC Jr, Moore SB. Transfusion-related acute lung injury: A neglected, serious complication of hemotherapy. Transfusion 1992;32:589-92.

15. Popovsky MA, Davenport RD. Transfusion-related acute lung injury: Femme fatale? Transfusion 2001;41:312-15.

16. Insunza A, Romon I, Gonzalez-Ponte ML, et al. Implementation of a strategy to prevent TRALI in a regional blood centre. Transfus Med 2004;14:157-64.

17. Engelfriet CP, Reesnik HW. International Forum: Transfusion-related acute lung injury (TRALI). Vox Sang 2001;81:269-83.

18. Transfusion-related acute lung injury. Association bulletin #05-09. Bethesda, MD: AABB, 2005. [Available at http://www.aabb.org/Content/Members_Area/Association_Bulletins/ab05-9.htm (accessed July 3, 2008).]

19. Kleinman S. A perspective on transfusion-related acute lung injury two years after the Canadian Consensus Conference (editorial). Transfusion 2006;46:1465-8.

20. Kleinman S, Caulfield T, Chan P, et al. Toward an understanding of transfusion-related acute lung injury: Statement of a consensus panel. Transfusion 2004;44:1774-89.

21. Transfusion-related acute lung injury. Association bulletin #06-07. Bethesda, MD: AABB, 2006. [Available at http://www.aabb.org/Content/Members_Area/Association_Bulletins/ab06-07.htm (accessed July 3, 2008).]

22. Bux J, Sachs UJH. The pathogenesis of transfusion-related acute lung injury (TRALI). Br J Haematol 2007;136:788-99.

23. Bux J. Transfusion-related acute lung injury (TRALI): A serious adverse event of blood transfusion. Vox Sang 2005;89:1-10.

24. Silliman CC, Ambruso DR, Boskov LK. Transfusion-related acute lung injury. Blood 2005;105:2266-73.

25. Engelfriet CP, Reesnik HW. International Forum: Measures to prevent TRALI. Vox Sang 2007;92:258-77.

26. Clarifications to recommendations to reduce the risk of TRALI. Association bulletin #07-03. Bethesda, MD: AABB, 2007. [Available at http://www.aabb.org/Content/Members_Area/Association_Bulletins/ab07-03.htm (accessed July 3, 2008).]

27. Rebulla P, Finazzi G, Marangoni F, et al. The threshold for prophylactic platelet transfusion in adults with acute myeloid leukemia. N Engl J Med 1997;337:1870-5.

28. Wandt H, Frank M, Ehninger G, et al. Safety and cost effectiveness of a 10×10^9/L trigger for prophylactic platelet transfusions compared with the traditional 20×10^9/L trigger: A prospective comparative trial in 105 patients with acute myeloid leukemia. Blood 1998;91:3601-6.

29. Heckman KD, Weiner GJ, Davis CS, et al. Randomized study of prophylactic platelet transfusion threshold during induction therapy for adult acute leukemia: 10,000/μL versus 20,000/μL. J Clin Oncol 1997;15:1143-9.

30. Zumberg MS, del Rosario MLU, Nejame CF, et al. A prospective randomized trial of prophylactic platelet transfusion and bleeding incidence in hematopoietic stem cell transplant recipients: 10,000/μL versus 20,000/μL trigger. Biol Blood Marrow Transplant 2002;8:569-76.

31. Freireich EJ, Kliman A, Gaydos LA, et al. Response to repeated platelet transfusion from the same donor. Ann Intern Med 1963;59:277-87.

32. Djerassi I, Farber S, Evans AE. Transfusions of fresh platelet concentrates to patients with secondary thrombocytopenia. N Engl J Med 1963;268:221-6.

33. McVay PA, Toy PT. Lack of increased bleeding after paracentesis and thoracentesis in patients with mild coagulation abnormalities. Transfusion 1991;21: 164-71.

34. McVay PA, Toy PT. Lack of increased bleeding after liver biopsy in patients with mild hemostatic abnormalities. Am J Clin Pathol 1990;94:747-53.

35. Bishop JF, Schiffer CA, Aisner J, et al. Surgery in acute leukemia: A review of 167 operations in thrombocytopenic patients. Am J Hematol 1987;26:147-55.

36. Practice parameter for the use of fresh-frozen plasma, cryoprecipitate, and platelets. Development Task Force of the College of American Pathologists. JAMA 1994;271:777-81.

37. Stroncek DF, Rebulla P. Transfusion medicine 2: Platelet transfusions. Lancet 2007;370:427-38.

38. Segal JB, Dzik WH. Paucity of studies to support that abnormal coagulation test results predict bleeding in the setting of invasive procedures: An evidence-based review. Transfusion 2005;45:1413-25.

39. Stanworth SJ, Brunskill SJ, Hyde CJ, et al. Is fresh frozen plasma clinically effective? A systematic review of randomized controlled trials. Br J Haematol 2004;126:139-52.

40. Practice parameters for use of red blood cell transfusions. College of American Pathologists. Arch Pathol Lab Med 1998;122:130-8.

41. British Committee for Standards in Haematology Blood Transfusion Task Force. Guidelines for the clinical use of red cell transfusions. Br J Haematol 2001;133:24-31.

42. Klein HG, Spahn DR, Carson JL. Transfusion medicine 1: Red blood cell transfusion in clinical practice. Lancet 2007;370:415-25.

43. Hébert P, Wells G, Blajchman MA, et al. A multicenter randomized controlled clinical trial of transfusion requirements in critical care. N Engl J Med 1999; 340:409-17.

44. Lacroix J, Hébert PC, Hutchison JS, et al. Transfusion strategies for patients in pediatric intensive care units. N Engl J Med 2007;356:1609-19.

45. Bracey AW, Radovancevic R, Riggs SA, et al. Lowering the hemoglobin threshold for transfusion in coronary artery bypass procedures: Effect on patient outcome. Transfusion 1999;39:1070-7.

46. Rao SV, Jollis JG, Harrington RA, et al. Relationship of blood transfusion and clinical outcomes in patients with acute coronary syndromes. JAMA 2004; 292:1555-62.

47. Wu WC, Rathore SS, Wang Y, et al. Blood transfusion in elderly patients with acute myocardial infarction. N Engl J Med 2001;345:1230-6.
48. Carson JL, Terrin ML, Magaziner J, et al. Transfusion trigger trial for functional outcomes in cardiovascular patients undergoing surgical hip fracture repair (FOCUS). Transfusion 2006;36:2192-206.
49. Katz LM, Kiss JE. Plasma for transfusion in the era of transfusion-related acute lung injury mitigation. Transfusion 2008;48:393-7.
50. Riedler GF, Haycox AR, Duggan AK, Dakin HA. Cost-effectiveness of solvent/detergent-treated fresh-frozen plasma. Vox Sang 2003;85:88-95.
51. Sachs UJH, Kauschat D, Bein G. White blood-cell reactive antibodies are undetectable in solvent/detergent plasma. Transfusion 2005;45:1628-31.
52. Renaudier P, Vo Mai M, Ounnoughene N, et al. Epidemiology of transfusion-related acute lung injury in e-FIT, the French hemovigilance database: 1994 to 2006 (abstract). Transfusion 2007;47(Suppl 3S):7A.
53. Sinnott P, Bodger S, Gupta A, Brophy M. Presence of HLA antibodies in single-donor-derived fresh frozen plasma compared with pooled, solvent detergent-treated plasma (Octaplas). Eur J Immunogenet 2004;31:271-4.
54. Salge-Bartels U, Breitner-Ruddock S, Hunfeld A, et al. Are quality differences responsible for different adverse reactions reported for SD-plasma from USA and Europe? Transfus Med 2006;16:266-75.
55. Silva MA, Gregory KR, Carr-Greer MA, et al. Summary of the AABB Interorganizational task force on bacterial contamination of platelets: Fall 2004 impact survey. Transfusion 2006;46:636-41.
56. Densmore TL, Goodnough LT, Ali S, et al. Prevalence of HLA sensitization in female apheresis donors. Transfusion 1999;39:103-6.
57. MacLennan S, Lucas G, Brown C, et al. Prevalence of HLA and HNA antibodies in donors: Correlation with pregnancy and transfusion history (abstract). Vox Sang 2004;87(Suppl 3):4.
58. Triulzi D, Kakaiya R, Schreiber G. Donor risk factors for white blood cell antibodies associated with transfusion-related acute lung injury: REDS Leukocyte Antibody Prevalence Study (LAPS) (editorial). Transfusion 2007;47:563-4.
59. Triulzi D, Kakaiya R, Kleinman S, et al. Relationship of HLA antibodies in blood donors to pregnancy and transfusion history (abstract). Transfusion 2007;47(Suppl 3S):2A.
60. Stroncek DF, Fadeyi E, Adams S. Leukocyte antigen and antibody detection assays: Tools for assessing and preventing pulmonary transfusion reactions. Transfus Med Rev 2007;21:273-86.
61. Lucas DP, Paparounis ML, Myers L, et al. Detection of HLA Class I specific antibodies by the QuickScreen enzyme linked immunosorbent assay. Clin Diagn Lab Immunol 1997;4:252-7.
62. Pei R, Wang C, Tarsitani S, et al. Simultaneous HLA Class I and Class II antibody screening with flow cytometry. Hum Immunol 1998;59:313-22.
63. Curtis BR, McFarland JG. Mechanism of transfusion-related acute lung injury (TRALI): Anti-leukocyte antibodies. Crit Care Med 2006;34(Suppl):S118-23.
64. Norris PJ, Gottschall JL, Lee JH, et al. Long-term persistence of anti-HLA antibodies and slightly enhanced detection using serum vs plasma (abstract). Transfusion 2006;46(Suppl):122A.

65. Lucas G, Rogers S, de Haas M, et al. Report on the Fourth International Granulocyte Immunology Workshop: Progress toward quality assessment. Transfusion 2002;42:462-8.

66. Clay M, Kline W, McCullough J. The frequency of granulocyte-specific antibodies in postpartum sera and a family study of the 6B antigen. Transfusion 1984;24:252-5.

67. Stroncek DE, Klein HG. Heavy breathing in the blood bank: Is it transfusion-related acute lung injury, our anxiety, or both? (editorial) Transfusion 2007;47:559-62.

68. Sachs UJ, Bux J. TRALI after transfusion of crossmatch-positive granulocytes. Transfusion 2003;43:1683-6.

69. O'Connor JC, Strauss RG, Goeken NE, Knox LB. A near-fatal reaction during granulocyte transfusion of a neonate. Transfusion 1988;28:173-6.

Index

M

Male-donor plasma program, 143-158
  clinical features and outcomes in,
    146-147
  conclusions of, 154-158
  implementation and effect of policy,
    104, 149-153, 163, 168
  implicated components in, 148-
    149
  overview of, 144-146, 171-172
  serologic findings in, 147-148
Massive transfusion, 16-20
Mixed passive agglutination assay, 131-
  132
Monoclonal antibody immobilization of
  neutrophil antigens assay (MAINA),
  131-132
Monocytes, 54, 61
Mortality rates, 5-6, 103, *145,* 161-163

N

Neutrophils. *See also* HNA antibodies;
  Human neutrophil antigens
  interplay with endothelial cells, 54
  isolation process for, 128, 130
  priming and activation of, 46, 50-
    52, *56*
  role in TRALI, 45-47
  transfusion of, 63, 121, 136
  transit through lungs, 47, 49
Nitric oxide, 29
Notification to donor, of HLA antibodies,
  179

O-P

Oxygen, supplemental, in treatment, 36
Pathogenesis of TRALI, 25-29
  biologic response modifiers in, 28-
    29
  leukocyte antibodies in, 26-28, 45-
    46
Pathophysiology of TRALI, 43-64
  leukocyte antibodies in, 45-46
  mechanisms leading to lung
    damage in, 50-55
  neutrophil transit through lungs in,
    47-49

priming and activating substances
  in, 55-63
  threshold model in, 46-47, *48*
Phenotyping neutrophil antigens, 133-
  134
Plasma components
  collected by apheresis, 172-173
  deferrals from donating, 74-78,
    137
  fatalities from, 103, 163
  from female donors
    minimizing use of, 103-104,
      163, 168
    of plasma collected by
      apheresis, 173
    of plasma manufactured from
      whole blood, 171-172
    and risk of TRALI, 24-25,
      148, *150,* 155
  guidelines for use of, 169-170
  implicated in TRALI, 86-89
  incidence of TRALI from, 7, *152*
  leukocyte antibodies in, 27-28, 45-
    46
  male-donor program for, 143-158
    clinical features and outcomes
      in, 146-147
    conclusions of, 154-158
    implementation and effect of
      policy for, 103, 149-153,
      163, 168
    implicated components in,
      148-149
    overview of, 144-146, 171-
      172
    serologic findings in, 147-148
  in massive transfusion, 20
  in pulmonary transfusion reactions,
    121
  and risk of ALI/ARDS, 20, 23-25,
    28
  and risk of TRALI, 148, *149-150,*
    151-152, *153,* 154-155, 163
  risk-reduction strategies for, 167,
    171-174
  solvent/detergent-treated (ie, FFP),
    151, 157, 173-174